MOVE YOURSELF

Happy

Move Yourself Happy
Dianne Buswell

First published in the UK and USA in 2023 by
Watkins, an imprint of Watkins Media Limited
Unit 11, Shepperton House, 83–93 Shepperton
Road, London N1 3DF

enquiries@watkinspublishing.com

Commissioning Editor: Anya Hayes
Managing Editor: Lucy Carroll
Assistant Editor: Brittany Willis
Text Development: Kate Latham
Copyeditor: Emma Hill
Head of Design: Karen Smith
Designer: Alice Claire Coleman
Production: Uzma Taj
Commissioned Photography: Katrina Lipska
Shoot Consultant: Sabrina Kelly
Hair and Makeup: Hannah Kreeger
   & Shari Rendle
Clothes Stylists: Harriet Byczok
   & Sue Mee Cheung

A CIP record for this book is available from the
British Library

ISBN: 978-1-78678-670-8 (Paperback)
ISBN: 978-1-78678-677-7 (eBook)

10 9 8 7 6 5 4 3 2 1

Printed in China

Publisher's note
While every care has been taken in compiling
the recipes for this book, Watkins Media
Limited, or any other persons who have
been involved in working on this publication,
cannot accept responsibility for any errors
or omissions, inadvertent or not, that may
be found in the recipes or text, nor for any
problems that may arise as a result of preparing
one of these recipes. If you are pregnant or
breastfeeding or have any special dietary
requirements or medical conditions, it is
advisable to consult a medical professional
before following any of the recipes contained
in this book.

Notes on the recipes
Unless otherwise stated:
Use medium fruit and vegetables
Use medium (US large) organic or free-range
eggs
Use fresh herbs, spices and chillies
Use granulated sugar (Americans can use
ordinary granulated sugar when caster sugar
is specified)
Do not mix metric, imperial and US cup
measurements:
1 tsp = 5ml 1 tbsp = 15ml 1 cup = 240ml

www.watkinspublishing.com

DIANNE BUSWELL

MOVE YOURSELF

Happy

21 Days to Make
Joyful Movement
a Habit

WATKINS
Sharing Wisdom
Since 1893

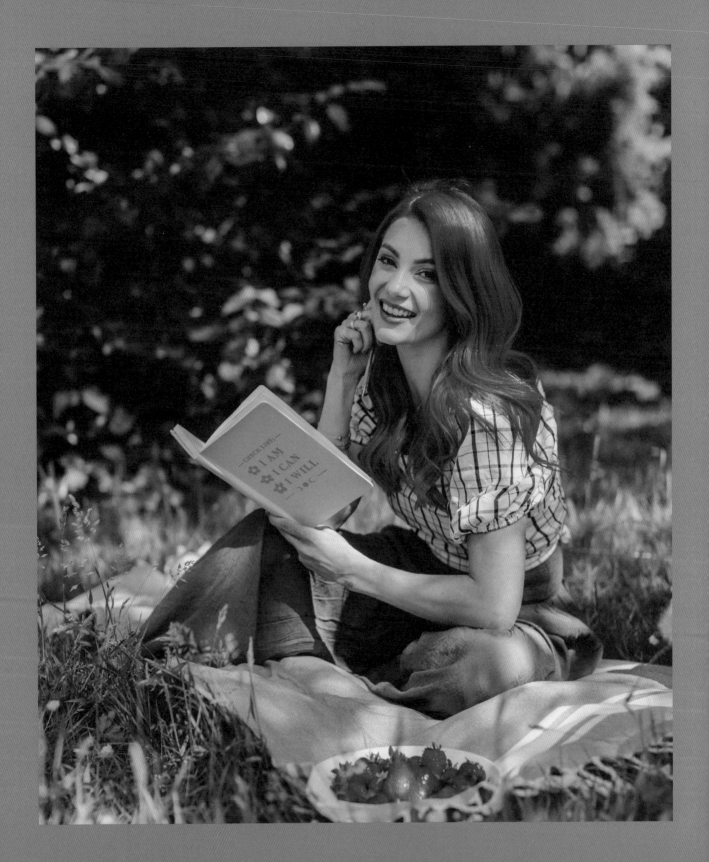

Contents

INTRODUCTION

Many people pick up a book on exercise because they want to get fit – perhaps they'd like to lose weight, fit back into their favourite jeans or look better for a party in a month's time. Exercise is so often about aesthetics, the superficial stuff – unless perhaps we've had a health scare or similar. We usually embark on a fitness or health kick when we have something negative going on, especially if we feel under pressure to change something about who we are or our bodies. When did you last think about putting on your running shoes or rolling out your yoga mat in order to have fun? To take care of your body? To feel good about yourself? That's what we've lost in our relationship with movement – it's become something we "have" to do.

Modern life takes movement away from us in so many ways – better transport options, sedentary screen-filled jobs and any products and takeaway meal we want delivered to our door. We've lost that connection with our natural movement – everything we need is within easy reach and movement so diminished in our lives.

As many of you know, I began dancing when I was young. I caught the bug and was lucky enough to make it my career, which means I get to do something I love every day and travel around the world. But what still gives me the biggest kick is teaching dance to others. It's the enjoyment they get from being caught up in the music, from challenging their body to discover completely new rhythms of movement, and achieving something they didn't think they could. Some find it easier than others, but everyone comes away from learning to dance with a new relationship with their body, and a whole new take on the power of movement to make you feel SO good, so alive and energized and with a whole host of health benefits on the side.

I want to show you that getting fit doesn't need to be about running marathons or "feeling the burn". You don't need to find two hours a day around work, family, kids and life to make a big difference to your health. I want to share the joy that movement gives, the buzz that ten minutes of getting active every day makes you feel, and how movement is at the heart of a healthy body and mind.

21 Days of Easy Wins to Get Movement into Your Day

I created the 21-Day Plan (see pages 149–202) to turn around your relationship with your body and movement, and to help you find the best exercise for you – exercise that you want to keep doing. I'll show you different ways to bring movement into your life and bolster that with lifestyle hacks and tips on nutrition, rest and fostering a positive mindset to make you feel great.

I've devised 21 fun and effective movement routines that will change your body and the way you feel about moving it. Whether you're tempted to try tap or salsa, body conditioning or ballet,

Pilates or a yoga flow, there is something for everyone, and it'll only take a few minutes every day. I've chosen three techniques that complement each other and that have been life-changing for me – yoga, Pilates and, of course, dance – that will put a big smile on your face.

In **Part 1: The Move Yourself Happy Way**, we're going to delve into the four key aspects of health that will nourish your body and mind, increase your flexibility, free you from aches and pains and leave you feeling energized and alive. **Part 2: The Movements** provides step-by-step guides to a range of simple and effective moves, poses and positions that introduce dance, Pilates and yoga in a fun and accessible way. **Part 3: 21 Days to a Stronger, Happier You** is where you can explore your relationship with movement and health, and try out 21 quick and uplifting dance, yoga and Pilates routines that I specially created for this book in order to help you create a whole new movement habit. Regular and consistent movement makes a difference – this is not about full-on HIIT sessions and fancy outfits; it's about getting real with your body and showing it the love it deserves. The plan also includes weekly mantras and journaling prompts to help promote a positive mindset, along with nutrition advice and delicious recipes to nurture your beautiful body.

You might not feel as if you have the energy to do this right now – but I PROMISE, give me 21 days and I'll have you sleeping better, moving freely and feeling fantastic about yourself. And there's no fancy equipment needed to make these changes; all of the routines are easy to do from the comfort of your own home.

THIS IS FOR YOU

This book is a guide, not gospel. You are you, and life is about finding out more about what you enjoy, and what makes you feel good in your own way. The real secret to health is finding the joy in movement, and then enjoying and appreciating what your body and mind get in return. Who wouldn't want more flexibility, co-ordination, balance, sleep and happiness?

Movement and exercise are at the beginning and the end of how I live my life. They give me the energy to work and play and to feel good about myself, and the more ways I find to enjoy movement and exercise, the more my life is filled with joy. I want the same for you.

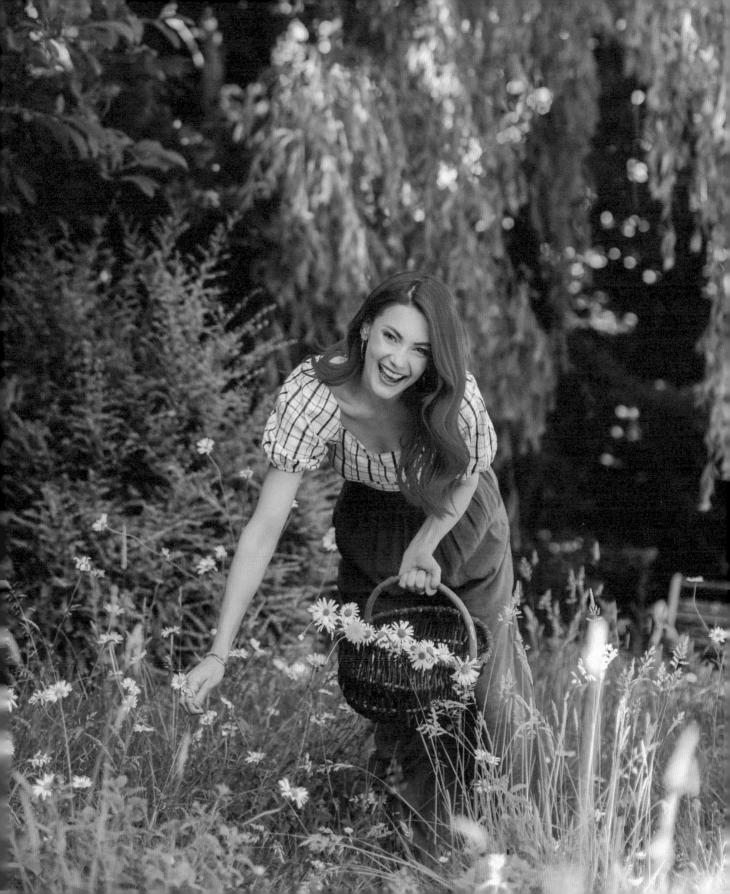

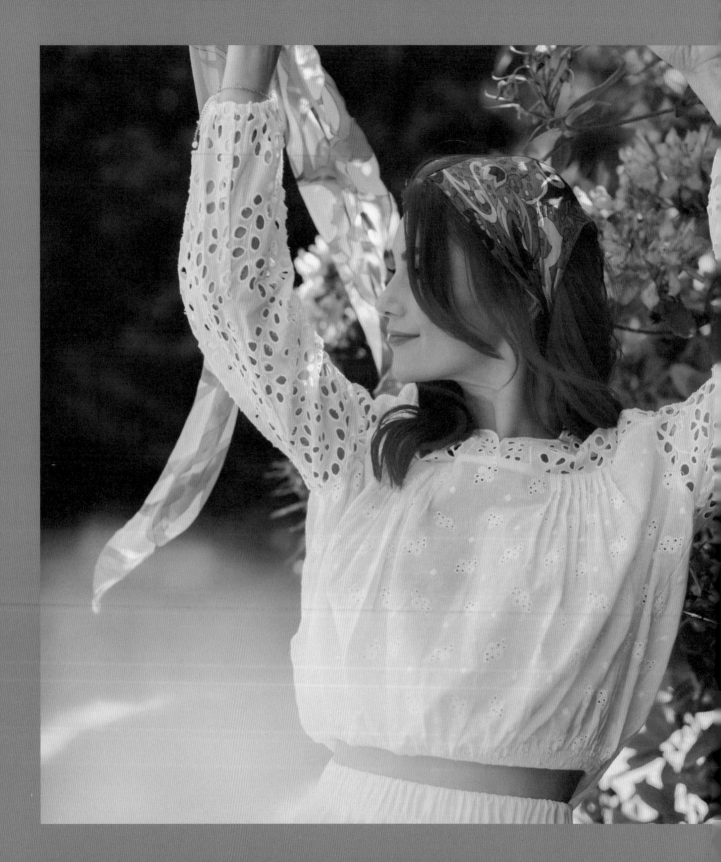

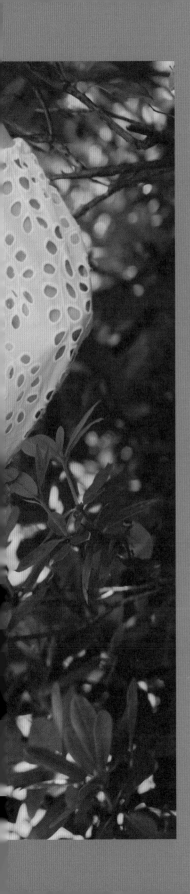

Part 1

The Move Yourself Happy Way

Before we look at the moves and routines we're going to be trying over the next three weeks, I want to talk about the Four Pillars of wellbeing that I follow to feel good. They are the cornerstones of living well and looking after yourself – self-care is at the heart of it all. Nourish yourself and you'll find it easier to get up in the morning, rise above stress and worry, and you'll have the energy to do everything you love. And I'm aiming to show you how you can achieve this with some simple tools and hacks – not by making life more complicated. You're worth it!

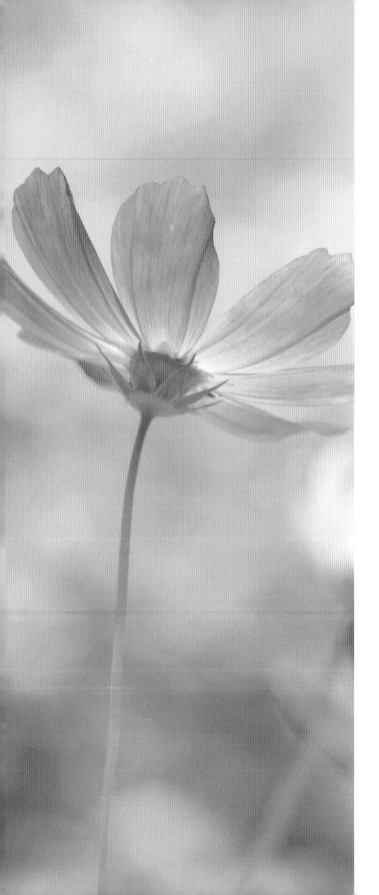

THE FOUR PILLARS OF STAYING HAPPY AND HEALTHY

Being a dancer can be tough, physically and mentally, so I've had to discover what works best to strengthen my body and mind, to enable me to perform consistently at a high level and to allow me to find balance in my life.

Dancing is certainly something that requires a healthy body – I found that out the hard way ...

There is a lot of pressure in the dancing world and the more successful I became in my career, the more pressure I felt to look a certain way and be the best on the dance floor. I'm pretty competitive and work hard at what I do. I was in my late twenties and comparing my body to the other dancers and those around me, working so hard to do my best and putting huge pressure on myself all the time. We all look different, and we dance in our own way with our own distinct personalities, but I felt so pressured to look like other dancers in order to keep my job and to "keep up".

It got to the point where I would do anything I could to try to lose weight – I tried lots of diets, I would skip meals or make myself sick. I stopped eating and really restricted myself. I'd eat an apple and then make myself work out afterwards to make up for it. The joy of movement was entirely lost for me.

It wasn't until I couldn't do what I loved that I realized how serious the situation was. At that time, I'd started to actually hate dancing – I just didn't have the energy for it. There was no part of me that looked forward to a show. I was so weak – even walking up a few stairs left me needing to stop because I was out of breath. Before a show, I would lock myself in a toilet and pray that I'd get through it as I wasn't sure I could. Performing became my worst nightmare – and that was the point at which I knew I couldn't physically or mentally carry on.

I made the decision to leave the show and I flew home. With the support of my family, I went straight to the doctors – and they called me back just a couple of hours later to say that I was dangerously low in iron and nutrients and I needed some immediate treatment. That was a huge blow and made me realize how bad things had become. Speaking to family really helped me and I knew that I wanted to get myself healthy again. I'd never not loved my dancing before, but it had become a chore or a punishment, and that made me realize how my body is my engine. In order to do what I loved, I needed to fuel my body, to give it nourishment and love. It was a life-changing turning point for me and my relationship with my body and my health.

You could say that, along with my family and friends, dance saved me. Some people keep on spiralling down, but I was lucky enough to be able to take myself out of the situation, so that I could talk to people and get help.

That's when I fell in love with the process of nourishing and caring for my body. I learned to enjoy a range of exercises, not just high intensity ones, and to allow my body to rest if it needed to. – which was another learning curve for me. I was so used to constantly working out and it had become rather an obsession, but having that break allowed me to enjoy movement again. I started with yoga – it was enjoyable and healing movement focused on time for myself and rest rather than a gruesome need to burn calories.

I'll never forget the first time I went back on stage after getting better – it was such an emotional moment. My body felt good – it was tingling and I had my old energy back. Just doing what I loved again was the best feeling ever.

The Four Pillars

I've become fascinated by the stories of those who live in the "Blue Zones" around the world – areas where communities seem to live healthier and longer on average than elsewhere in the world. The zones range from Okinawa in Japan in the East to Loma Linda in California in the West, via Greece, Italy and Costa Rica. At first glance, these communities lack a common thread, but research has shown certain lifestyle habits that cross cultures allow the average person to live a longer, healthier and happier life. Studies reveal that eating a largely plant-based diet focusing on natural wholefoods, plenty of natural movement and a positive mindset, all tied together with being part of a community and keeping social, are powerful components of longevity.

My own experiences have led me to understand that there are four key areas that I need to balance in my life to guarantee I am happy and healthy, energized and motivated. I know that my diet influences how I feel, that finding the time to focus on my mental health is hugely important and that taking time out for myself is crucial. These are the Four Pillars of my approach to wellbeing:

1. **Movement**: Let's move because we want to and because it makes us feel so good, rather than because we have to.
2. **Nutrition**: Eating well gives your body the nourishment and energy it needs to support your optimum physical and mental health – in a joyful way.
3. **Rest**: Even before movement, rest is at the core of finding balance and contentment in our lives, and is especially necessary for a successful relationship with exercise.
4. **Positivity**: Mental strength and a positive outlook is key to achieving what we want and supporting a balanced life.

The major positive that came out of what happened to me was that it became clear how important it is to protect and balance my mind and body.

I had been so off balance and unhappy, living at about 100 miles an hour, doing hours of training and performing and travelling while trying (and often failing) to fit friends and family around that. There was certainly no time for anything except work – no hobbies or downtime. I kept pushing myself and something had to give. The realization of the importance of self-care became a passion of mine after this, because I could see the immense impact ignoring it had on me. Often, we already know the things we need to do to take care of ourselves, but don't prioritize them.

21 Days to Create a Movement Habit

I devised the 21-Day Plan to help you to bring these Four Pillars into your life, to make movement a natural part of your day, to show you all the ways that exercise, nutrition, rest and a positive mindset can lift you up and power you through whatever life is throwing at you. And to prove to you that exercise can be your thing.

Perhaps you've never found your exercise groove and you do a bit of this and a little of that. Or you exercise for the sake of exercise, but haven't yet found the joy in doing so, and in reaping the benefits in all areas of your life. I've worked with those who are time-poor, energy-lacking or just don't feel that exercise if for them, but we all need to move our bodies for optimum health and mental wellbeing.

Research shows that 21 days is roughly how long it takes to create a new habit. It's never too late to make lasting change. Routine is the answer: exercise little and often and listen to how it makes you feel. Change your body and how it feels forever by discovering your own positive relationship with movement. Let's get moving and get happy!

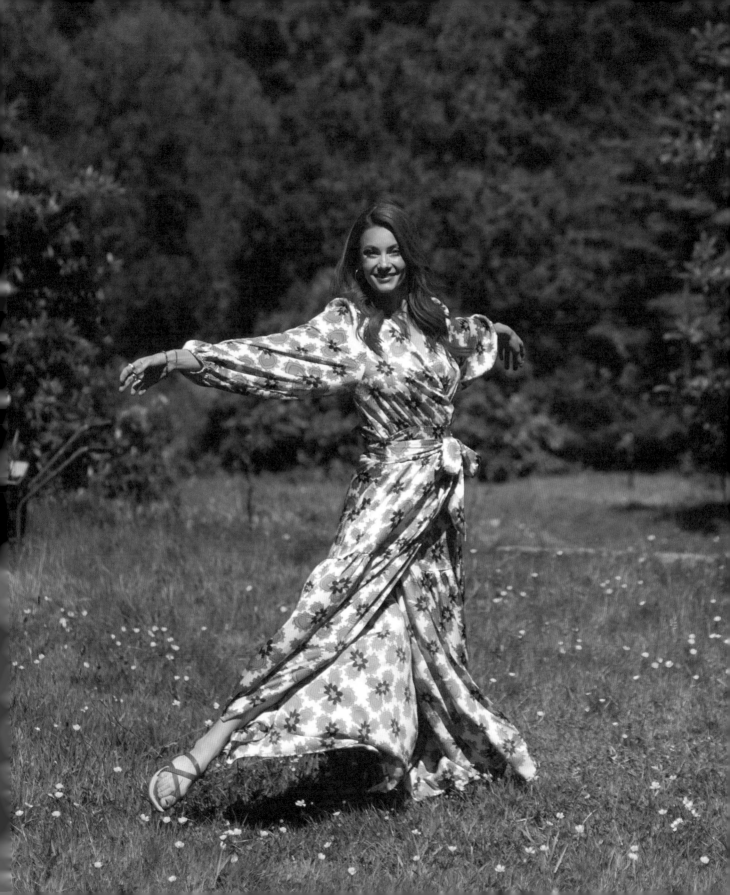

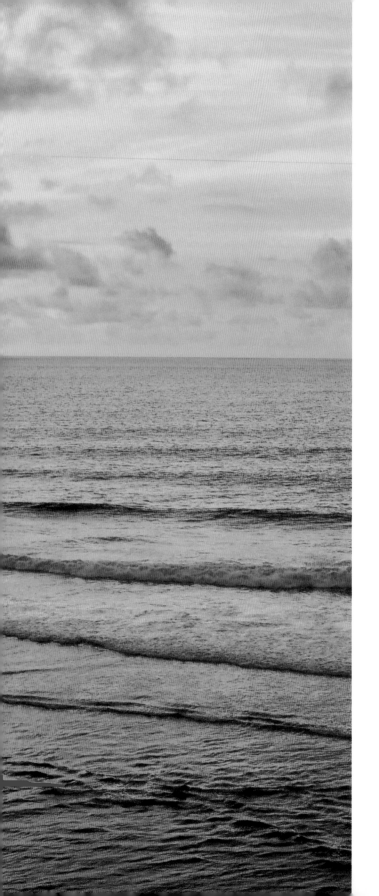

THE POWER OF MOVEMENT

I've been dancing from such a young age and finding joy in movement is something that was a saviour for me growing up.

Many people struggle to exercise – often they work out because they this and that about their body and their life. Exercise is a punishment, a thing to tick off a list of must-dos and should-dos, a chore that has to be done.

To me, the first pillar of a healthy lifestyle – movement – is about self-love. Exercise should be like going shopping or any of those other things we love that we make time for and look forward to. We should be saying, "I'm going to make time for this because I enjoy it." My relationship with movement began when I was young – I started dancing when I was about three years old. My older brother would take me along to his classes. He asked, "Do you want to come along?" one day and I just kept going. I come from Bunbury in Western Australia. It's a small town so not many boys were dancing, which meant I was lucky to find a partner and we began competing.

And I was obsessed with dance. I enjoyed the physicalness of the training, but it was the going out and performing that felt like the heartbeat of it all for me – dancing freely without the pressure of competition and "you're doing it right/wrong" – moving my body in that way made me so happy.

When I found yoga and Pilates later, they were a revelation for me – here were other ways of moving my body that were pure joy. I fell in love all over again with how movement made me feel, mentally and physically. They were another form of dance for me in a way, but with more emphasis on listening to my own body and breathing, plus the power of slow, controlled movement.

What was revelatory for me was the whole stillness part to yoga, which changed lots of aspects of my life as well as my dancing. Growing up I always thought that the more energy I put into dancing and movement, the better it would be – full-on all the way through. With yoga, I came to realize the importance of the still and calm parts of dance, that these were as beautiful and so necessary to allow the enjoyment and appreciation of the more energetic movement.

Exercise is Not Punishment

Yoga helped me to view the way I was living and working differently, and gave me permission to not always feel like I had to go, go, go. This changed the way I experienced things. With my dancing and rehearsing, it allowed me to step away from the peer pressure to constantly push myself and work to be something else. I understood about the necessity of listening to my own body, to do dancing my way, and about the connection of the body and mind.

Of course I'd heard the phrase "healthy body, healthy mind" plenty of times, but I wish someone had properly explained it to me when I was younger. I was always pushing myself to work harder, dance better, and looking at those around me and trying to be something else. I used to think the fitter I was, the better a dancer I would be, and that how I looked and the shape of my body were crucial. The dancing world can be tough that way. Now, when I look at someone dancing or even moving, I look at the expression they give to their dancing and the feeling it gives me.

Our Early Relationship with Movement

Growing up in Australia and living an outdoors lifestyle led me to naturally prioritize exercise from the start. I had two brothers as well. One of my brothers was the dancer, so I would go dancing with him and I would kick a ball around with my other brother. Then I would ask him to come play tennis with me. My friend played netball so I spent a lot of time doing that too. When you're young, you move a lot without even thinking about it – climbing in playgrounds, hanging off monkey bars and bouncing on trampolines. When does our constant desire to move stop? When does sitting become our default activity and our way to rest and wind down?

In Australia most kids I went to school with had a sport or active hobby, and that keeps a lot of people moving and enjoying movement regularly. A hobby or activity only takes a couple of hours each week, but you feel so good after making that time, physically and mentally. Getting active usually involves some socializing too and mixing with others – that community that is so important for us. So the activity becomes more of a thing you want to do because of the way you feel afterwards, and you keep going, whether you're good or not. It's the warm feelings inside and the laughter you share with others that make it fun.

Endorphins and Good Stuff

That buzz or high we get after being physically active comes from the chemicals that our bodies release when we get moving. We call them endorphins or "feel-good" chemicals and they act on our brains to release hormones such as dopamine that make us feel good (like when someone praises us). Research shows that these can also help with relieving stress and anxiety.

Of course we know that regular movement has an impact on our physical body too. It improves circulation and blood flow around the body, leading to a healthier heart, lungs, bones, muscles, brain function ... in fact, it enhances all our health systems. Becoming fitter leads to fewer aches and pains, which is also going to make us feel more positive.

Physical activity can be great for sleep too – it tires us out and helps reduce stress and worry. Better sleep also prompts a whole smorgasbord of positives for our mental and physical health. It's a win-win situation.

Incidental Movement

I want to shout from the rooftop that the good vibes that come with physical movement don't require us to run half-marathons every other day or push ourselves to the extreme. What our bodies need and relish is regular movement of all types, as part of our everyday life. So if you think of yourself as not a gym/running/cardio person, then that's fine. While getting a sweat on sometimes is good for our hearts, an hour of gardening and mowing the lawn is beneficial in so many ways too. Nike's mission statement says that "If you have a body, you are an athlete" – a powerful reminder of our body's potential.

Exercise that is good for us is too often billed as hard and it's implied that if you're having fun, then it's not real exercise. Movement is often done for the sake of exercise, a punishment that we have to get through and endure for the sake of our waistline or weight, when what we actually need is simply to get moving more and be positive about that.

Incidental exercise is the movement we do during the day that we don't think about – going up and down the stairs four times in five minutes when we can't find the car keys, walking the dog or running for the train. This is the sort of movement that is good for us, and it's free and easy to access.

Think back to the Blue Zones – those inhabitants have naturally physical lifestyles. Their main exercise is taken when going about their daily lives – doing the shopping, mopping the floor, meeting up with friends and family. They just get out and about.

We live very convenient lives these days. Food is delivered straight to our door. We want to do our shopping in just one store so that it takes less time and steps. Our meals take three minutes in the microwave (or are delivered to the door) rather than involving an hour of picking vegetables from the garden then pottering in the kitchen cooking

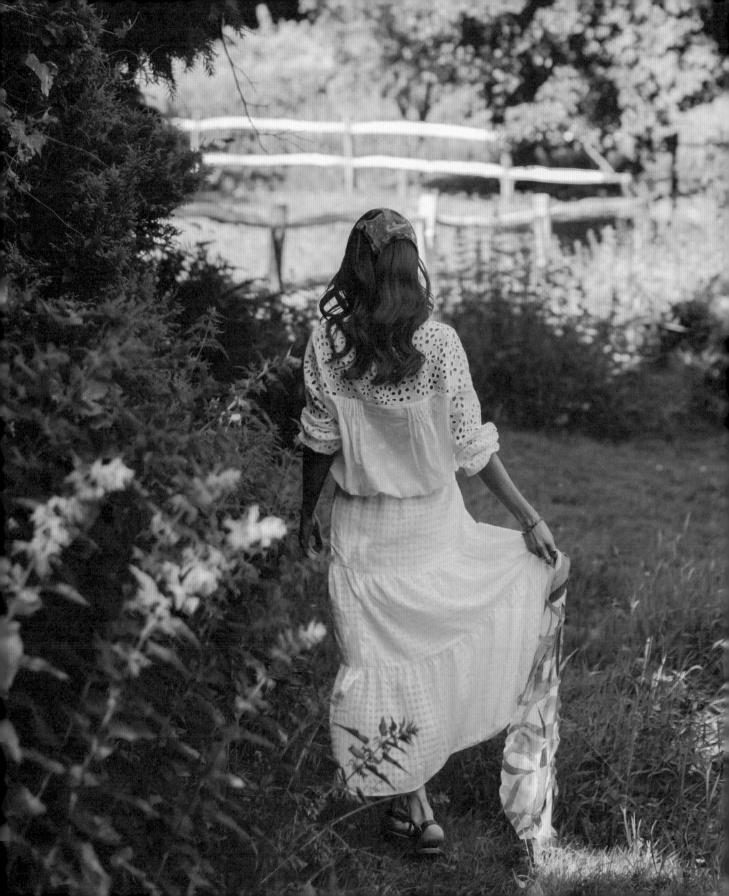

them up and making something special. All our labour-saving devices are actually movement-saving devices – from the remote control to the dishwasher. All these conveniences reduce movement to something that we have to sign up to do rather than it being a natural part of our day, and that has a huge impact on the level of exercise in our lives.

Just Start Moving

The best way to feel the benefit of moving more is just to start – that's the hardest part. I try to get in different forms of exercise each week – yoga, Pilates, some cardio and, of course, dancing. I'm generally always busy, so I plan my exercise in my diary to ensure that I do it and that I prioritize it – for my mental and physical happiness.

Doing an hour at the gym or a yoga class makes me feel so good, but one of my greatest feelings comes when every morning I take my coffee and walk around the garden for five minutes. That is such a good time for me. As I breathe in the fresh air, listen to the birds and look at what's growing in my garden, instantly my mood changes. I'm taking in the natural light and enjoying nature as I walk around when I would otherwise be sitting down, maybe watching the news, which can be a little triggering at times, and distracted by planning for the day ahead.

I notice that after I do this in the morning, I come back inside and am so much more ready for the day, feeling alive and energetic. This is just one of the small adjustments I make to bring energy and movement into my day – it might seem like nothing, but I know how significant it is for my body and mind at the start of the day.

Also, if I can walk somewhere I do, rather than take a car. I find these easy sort of adjustments, little things you can slot into the day, are great for effortlessly moving the body more. We're not made to be sat down for so many hours of the day, so we need to look for ways to move if our lives and jobs are not physically active.

Try to build in regular exercise to your week. Dust off your old skipping rope, put on a podcast and go for a walk in nature, or find a yoga class to do with a friend. Plan for how you can increase positive movement in your life – in five-minute bursts or longer sessions.

Find the Joy

Think about when you last felt joyful about movement. Perhaps you were swimming on holiday or riding a horse, shooting hoops with the kids or enjoying a hike with a friend.

Exercise needs to fit into your life, to be enjoyable and achievable. This isn't about getting a gym pass that you'll use four times then stop going. Take the time to think about what will make you happy and feel good. What does your body need at this time? Don't pressure yourself to be someone you're not – your friend might love running but if it's not right for you, or doesn't work right now, then that's fine. Exercise for you. For example, yesterday I was tired so I just did a few stretches. It is about listening to your body and recognizing the importance of movement in everyday life.

Exercise as Self-Care

As part of finding your own way to enjoy movement, I want you to view it as self-care. It's something we need in our lives to nourish ourselves, inside and out. If we make it less about what we "should" do, that frees us to enjoy the positives. I love my Pilates class and finding ten minutes each day for some yoga. I look forward to that time – it's me-time, when I can be in a relaxing environment, put aside any worries and concentrate on my body and me. At home, I might light a candle and put on relaxing or upbeat music. I want movement to feel like a spa moment – a time to put myself first.

It was the enjoyment that came with movement that first captivated me – for me and for others. The more I did it, the more I wanted to perform for people and make them happy when they watched me dancing on stage. It was my happy moment, my happy place. Let's find your movement happy place.

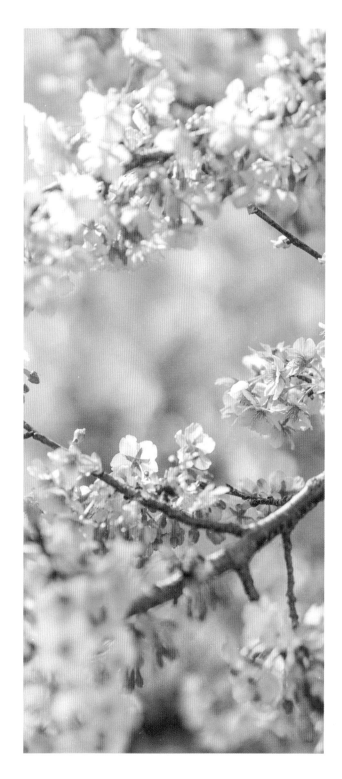

> "Take the time to think about what will make you happy and feel good. What does your body need?"

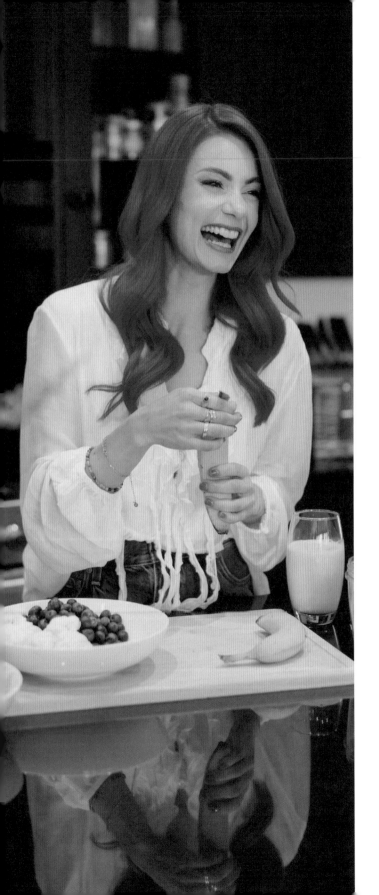

THE POWER OF NUTRITION

I love food and it's a massive part of my life. Most importantly, I'm not afraid to enjoy my food. What we put into our bodies is super-important – as crucial to our energy and mood as exercise. It needs to be part of our approach to moving our body: what we put in dictates what we get out, as I learned the hard way.

I have always found joy in cooking for others and sharing good food. My mum is Italian and that definitely influenced the family growing up – there is nothing I like better than to get together with loved ones for a family meal.

I cook lots at home and have done since I was young. Mum's a very good cook and taught me a lot about cooking techniques and using diverse ingredients. Growing up, she used such a range of fruits, vegetables and spices in the meals she cooked – plenty that weren't common then. There were also fantastic Italian dishes that her great-grandma had cooked that had been passed down – and she would tell me the "secret ingredients" that made them special. Now, one of my sisters-in-law is Filipino so she makes amazing Filipino food, and my other sister-in-law is Polish/Swedish and cooks great food with different tastes and combinations.

And then I have some people that I follow as well – some really good Instagram/YouTube accounts, such as @thefoodmedic and @georgieeatsuk.

Both of my brothers are gluten- and lactose-intolerant so mum had to adapt her cooking style when we were growing up. She now cooks a lot of dairy- and gluten-free dishes so I've learned classic Italian plus the gluten-free and the lactose-free versions, understanding and trialling substitutions. So food was definitely a huge part of growing up and is still a major part of my life.

Three Top Tips for Eating Well

I'm an open book when it comes to food. I enjoy trying new tastes and was never a fussy eater as a child. As I've talked about, I lost that for a while when I felt pressured to look a certain way. Now, being able to enjoy food that makes me feel good and gives me the strength and energy for my dancing is based on three key principles:

1. I've taken my eating **back to basics**. I eat as much natural food as possible – wholefoods without added extras – avoiding artificial preservatives and additives and packaged foods loaded with salt, sugar and trans fats. I don't want to over-complicate my diet but I want to know exactly what I'm putting in my body – foods that pass my "ingredients label test" (where all the ingredients are real foods and herbs and spices – not non-natural extras that I can't even pronounce).

2. We are all **bio-individual**. Certain foods will be "poison" to some people and amazing for others. Don't look at someone else's plate and think you should be eating what they're eating. This is one reason why diets, cutting out certain food groups and following eating restrictions aren't helpful ways to get healthy. Everyone's bodies and the ways we respond to foods are different. Find out what works for your body and nourish it.

3. **Crowding out** – rather than trying to eat less processed or unnatural food, fill your plates and meal plans with wholefoods. That way it's not about eating less of something, it's about consuming more nutrition-dense foods. Prioritize fruit, vegetables, protein and healthy carbs for meals and snacks and, nine times out of ten, without even thinking about it you're not going to feel a need for biscuits or crisps afterwards. It's not taking anything out, it's adding things in. Psychologically it works – rather than thinking that you need to cut things out and deprive yourself, you're crowding out your plate and feeling full and satisfied, so you don't have time to eat less healthy options. Don't take away, add!

These three tips help me achieve positive eating that reflects how my body feels and what it needs. I want to enjoy eating and cooking – and it doesn't stop me having a pizza or chocolate if that is what I want. It's all about moderation and powering my body.

Food for Energy

When I was young, I knew so little about nutrition. It wasn't until I started to struggle with my energy levels while I was dancing that I realized I needed to change something up. The connection between what you're putting into your body compared to what you're getting out is not always obvious.

In my early teen years, I was dancing at a high level and competing in competitions. I was doing so much exercise and dancing and thought that anything with sugar in it would be good as I needed the energy. So if I was going to a competition, I would take a packet of sweets or an energy drink and maybe some bananas. That would be all I'd have in a day when I would be dancing from morning to night, and I'd wonder why I couldn't sustain my energy levels. I'd start well but as the day went on, I'd feel tired and my dancing would suffer. I could feel the slump. I decided to try changing my diet and immediately noticed on those big competition days that eating differently gave me energy from start to finish – that was when I first saw the connection between eating well and the effects it had on my performance, energy and mood. I was blown away by how my body could feel so different just by changing something relatively simple in my diet.

Instead of taking sugary snacks and an energy drink on competition days, I (and my mum) would prep food ahead and I'd eat quite often during the day. I'd snack on homemade foods where I could name all the ingredients going into it – like nuts and fruit and wholegrains (and I'd still take the bananas). When I looked at the label on an energy drink and didn't recognize anything in it, I swapped that for a soluble vitamin drink.

Taking out the refined sugar and replacing it with wholefoods was a big deal at that young age – but the changes I felt in my body and my dancing on those long dancing days were irrefutable. I needed energy and to feel good when I was performing. When I switched up my eating habits, I suggested my dance partner, Kane, try a change too on the tough dancing days and he also saw a major difference.

Snack Well

Naturally when I'm working out and dancing more, I need more fuel for my body. I'm constantly hungry because my body is just chewing up energy. Working on shows all day every day, and dancing from 8am till 8pm, requires me to be super-prepared and feed my body regularly. It's about managing my energy levels – that's when it's crucial that I listen to my body. I definitely eat more during those times in comparison to when I'm not dancing, when my body naturally doesn't feel as hungry. It's worth remembering that snacking is a relatively modern thing – largely propelled by the mega snack food industry; don't fall into the trap of thinking they're always necessary.

Snacks can be especially difficult to keep healthy – it's easy to reach for a biscuit or something from a packet. When preparing a meal, you're more likely to choose a combination of protein, healthy carbs and vegetables, but snacking is where people fall down, grabbing the quick sugary option. The trick is to find easy ideas that work for your body and do you good.

I always prep some snacks to take with me for long days. If I have an early start dancing, after an hour I can be ready for my first snack of the day. Some of my favourite snacks are:

- Yogurt bark (see my recipe on this page)
- Rice cakes with peanut butter
- Crackers and cheese
- Vegetable sticks with a homemade dressing (I make my own easy citrus dressing – see page 29)
- Nuts and seeds
- Fruit – apples and bananas are easy to eat quickly
- Yogurts
- Dried fruit

I shop for ingredients in local specialist food shops and international aisles in the supermarket and buy in bulk – or I buy one extra special ingredient each week at the supermarket – to build up a stock of extras for recipes.

Here are some simple and delicious snack recipes that I wanted to share with you:

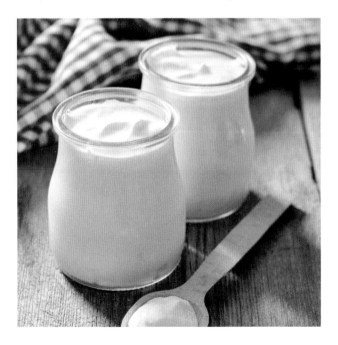

HOME-FLAVOURED YOGURT (SERVES 1)

Ingredients:
- 200ml (6¾fl oz) natural yogurt (or soy or coconut yogurt)
- 1 tsp grated orange zest
- Splash of orange juice
- Drop of vanilla extract
- Dash of honey or maple syrup
- Sprinkle of ground cinnamon

Method:
Mix all your ingredients together in a bowl. Enjoy chilled, straight from the refrigerator.

YOGURT BARK (MAKES 4–8 SNACK-SIZED SERVINGS)

Ingredients:
- 200ml (6¾fl oz) Home-Flavoured Yogurt (see recipe above)
- Handful of mixed berries, mixed seeds and chopped nuts (choose your favourites)
- Handful of goji berries
- 100g (3½oz) dark chocolate, chopped

Method:
Smear your flavoured yogurt over some baking paper on a baking sheet. Sprinkle with your choice of toppings. Melt the dark chocolate and drizzle over the top. Place in the freezer. Once frozen, break it up into snack-sized servings. I love experimenting with different toppings for this one.

RICE CAKE ROCKY ROAD (MAKES 8–10 SNACK-SIZED SERVINGS)

Ingredients:
- 6 plain rice cakes
- 100g (3½oz) walnuts, chopped
- 50g (1¾oz) goji berries
- Handful of frozen blueberries
- 1 tbsp peanut butter
- 60ml ((2fl oz) natural yogurt
- 100g (3½oz) dark chocolate, melted

Method:
Break up the rice cakes into a bowl and add your nuts and berries. Mix together, then add your peanut butter and yogurt. Pour into a shallow cake tin, drizzle the melted chocolate on top and refrigerate until hard. Cut into snack-sized portions. You can try a range of healthy additions for different flavours.

Prep Food for Fast Food

For meals as well as snacks, prepping ahead is the key to eating well and enjoying nourishing food when you don't have loads of time on your hands. I'm busy – like most people – and find that nutrition goes out of the window first when I am exhausted and trying to get the quickest and easiest fuel into my body.

Fast foods are often not good for us – they tend to come in packets with hidden preservatives, sugars and salt. Try to be organized and prep for the day or the week ahead whenever possible – it saves time on busy days. Use a quieter day or a weekend to put together snacks or meals and refrigerate or freeze them, then simply take them out as you need. I love a good prep session on a weekend to set me up for the week ahead – it makes me feel really smug! If I do a few dishes together, I save all that time and more during the week. Or get into the habit of making an extra portion of two of a meal every time you cook – you'll soon build up a stash of freezer options, or you'll be able to enjoy a healthy leftovers lunch with no extra work.

I Love Breakfast!

When I wake up, I like to start my day straight away. I wake up early and hungry so I can't wait to have my breakfast. I love oatmeal and add extras that will set me up for the day. Rolled oats are great for slow-release energy, and I might add in toppings for a nutrient-boost – favourites are prunes, goji berries, flaxseed or turmeric powder. I experiment with different milks, fruits, nuts, spices, as well as a variety of superfoods. Then I'm already ticking off some of my five-a-day.

Homemade granola, breakfast bowls or even a smoothie are such a good way to start the day and are great vegan options – plus they enable you to easily add a bunch of nutritious extras. There are so many options to bring in new flavours and fruits to this key meal – variety is great for your body and gut. I find that a good first meal of the day makes a big difference to how I feel for the rest of the day.

> "Prepping ahead is the key to eating well and enjoying nourishing food."

CHOCOLATE GRANOLA (SERVES 1-2)

Ingredients:

- 100g (3½oz) rolled oats
- 1 tsp cacao powder
- ¼ tsp ground cinnamon
- 1 tbsp coconut oil, melted
- 2 tbsp almond butter (or peanut butter)
- 1 tbsp maple syrup, honey or agave nectar
- Handful of dark chocolate chips or dark chocolate, grated (optional)

Method:

This homemade chocolate granola is better than any packaged chocolate cereal! Just mix together all of the ingredients, except the chocolate chips, spread out on a small baking tray and bake in the oven at 180°C (350°F) for about 20 minutes, stirring halfway through. Once cooled, mix in the chocolate chips or grate some dark chocolate (I use 100 per cent dark chocolate) on top, if using. This is such a treat of a breakfast.

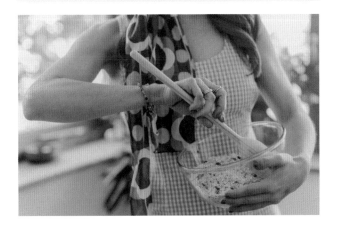

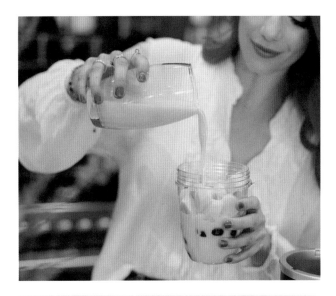

SUPER BREAKFAST SMOOTHIE #1 (SERVES 1)

Ingredients:

- Handful of frozen blueberries
- Handful of frozen cauliflower (This gives an extra boost of nutrients and it makes the smoothie creamy)
- 1 frozen banana
- About 75ml (2½fl oz) almond milk
- 1 tbsp almond butter
- Splash of lemon juice
- 1 tsp cacao powder
- 1 tsp maca powder

Method:

Simply whizz together all your ingredients in a blender. Smoothies are a great way to get your nutrients if breakfast is not really your thing. Try combinations of different fruits and milks to see what works for you.

SUPER BREAKFAST SMOOTHIE #2
(SERVES 1)

Ingredients:

- 1 frozen banana
- 2 pitted dates
- 1 tsp maple syrup or honey
- 1 tbsp rolled oats
- Pinch of ground cinnamon
- About 2 tbsp oat milk

Method:

Whizz all your ingredients together in a blender. Add as much oat milk as you need to achieve your preferred thickness. I love this sweet smoothie – it tastes luxurious.

QUINOA BREAKFAST BOWL (SERVES 1)

Ingredients

- 65g (2⅓oz) uncooked quinoa
- 235ml (8fl oz) almond milk
- 1 cinnamon stick
- 3 drops of vanilla extract

Method:

Place all your ingredients in a pan and simmer gently for 15 minutes, stirring occasionally. Remove the cinnamon stick and either serve this protein-packed start to your day straight away or keep in the fridge and serve cold or reheated the next morning. You can always add extra toppings too – blueberries, raspberries and chopped nuts are lovely.

I Don't Diet

Forget about any diet that you've ever heard of. I don't restrict myself in terms of what I can and cannot eat. I don't believe in having a "cheat day" or a "cheat meal." If I don't restrict myself, I find I'm not thinking about food so much because I know I can have it as I need. Telling myself I can't have something just makes it more attractive and I want those foods more.

Chocolate is something I always have around, but because I don't really eat so much sugary food anymore, my taste buds have changed – I enjoy dark chocolate but don't tend to want a lot of it. I used to love white chocolate or Dairy Milk as a kid, but now that level of sweetness is not a thing for me. Changing your diet will affect the food you want to eat – you actually crave fewer unhealthy options.

Again, "crowding out" my day with healthy food choices really is the best thing I do for my body and health. I think of it as going back to basics – back to when the fast food or processed food options weren't available.

Crowding Out

During the day, I take every opportunity to pack my meals full of vegetables and legumes. After a good breakfast and some healthy snacks, I might have a bean salad or wrap for lunch. The high protein and fibre content of the beans keep me full for longer. Or I might have a baked sweet potato with beans and cheese. Adding a handful of leaves, some tomatoes or a side salad means I get more vegetables as well. Using different dressings is a great way to liven up a lunchtime salad. Here are three of my favourite dressings, along with some of my go-to lunch options:

EASY CITRUS DRESSING (SERVES 1)

Ingredients:
- 1 tbsp lemon or lime juice
- 1 tbsp tahini
- Dash of light soy sauce
- Dash of olive oil
- Chilli flakes, to taste (optional)
- Salt and pepper for seasoning

Method:
Mix all the ingredients together in a small jug or bowl. I don't usually measure ingredients – just adjust for your taste buds. Test and adapt.

YOGURT DRESSING (SERVES 1)

Ingredients:
- 1 tbsp natural yogurt
- Squeeze of garlic paste
- Dash of lemon juice
- Dash of olive oil
- Chilli flakes, to taste (optional)
- Salt and pepper for seasoning

Method:
Mix all the ingredients together in a small jug or bowl. Drizzle over your favourite salad leaves.

> "Changing your diet will affect the food you want to eat – you actually crave fewer unhealthy options."

AVOCADO DRESSING (SERVES 1)

Ingredients:
- Flesh of ½ ripe avocado
- Dash of olive oil
- Splash of water
- Juice of 1 lemon
- Squeeze of garlic paste
- Handful of snipped chives
- Salt and pepper for seasoning

Method:
Blend together all the ingredients. This is a particular favourite mixed into a quinoa salad.

GREEK CHICKPEA SALAD (SERVES 1)

Ingredients:
- 2 handfuls of cooked chickpeas/ garbanzo beans (baked for extra crunch)
- Handful of pitted olives (any colour)
- Handful of chopped tomatoes
- Handful of chopped cucumber
- Handful of chopped red onion
- 100g (3½oz) feta cheese, diced (optional)

Method:
Combine your ingredients in a bowl, then add one of the dressings on this page, or a simple olive oil, lemon juice and dried oregano (plus salt and pepper) combo.

CHAR-GRILLED VEGGIE SALAD (SERVES 2–3)

Ingredients:

- ½ aubergine/eggplant, chopped
- 1 red or yellow pepper, deseeded and chopped
- ½ courgette/zucchini, chopped
- ½ butternut squash, deseeded and chopped
- 2–3 handfuls of cooked chickpeas/ garbanzo beans (optional)
- Olive or rapeseed oil
- Salt and pepper for seasoning
- Handful of quinoa or couscous, to serve

Method:

Toss your veg with the oil in a roasting tin and season. Add herbs or spices of your choice. Roast your veg at 190˚C (350˚F) for 25 minutes. At the same time, choose a grain to accompany the vegetables – such as couscous or quinoa – and cook according to the packet instructions. Serve with one of the dressings on page 29.

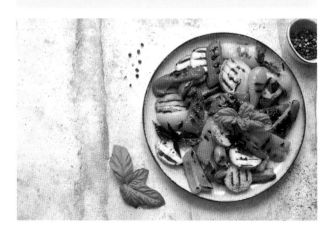

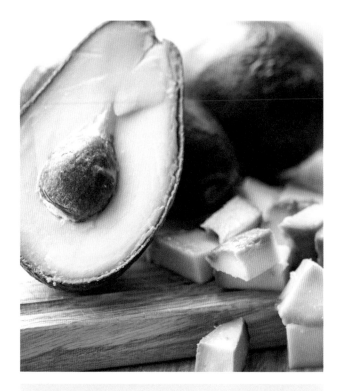

TUNA-STUFFED AVOCADO (SERVES 1)

Ingredients:

- 1 × 80g (2¾oz) can of tuna in brine, drained
- 1 tbsp mayonnaise
- Pinch of mustard seeds
- 1 celery stalk, chopped
- 2 spring onions/scallions, sliced
- ½ ripe avocado, stoned
- Salt and pepper for seasoning

Method:

Mix together the tuna, mayo, mustard seeds, celery, spring onions and salt and pepper and fill the avocado half. You can make it vegetarian by replacing the tuna with cooked quinoa.

EASY SWEET POTATO CHILLI
(SERVES 1)

Ingredients:
- 1 sweet potato
- ½ x 400g (14oz) can of four bean mix, drained
- 1 tsp chipotle paste
- 100ml (3⅓fl oz) vegetable stock
- Pinch of ground cumin
- Chilli flakes (to taste)
- 1 tbsp natural yogurt (optional)

Method:
Bake the sweet potato in the oven at 180°C (350°F) for about 40 minutes. Meanwhile, add the beans and other ingredients, except the yogurt, to a pan and warm through until thickened. Once cooked, cut open the potato and pour the bean chilli over it. Serve with a dollop of natural yogurt.

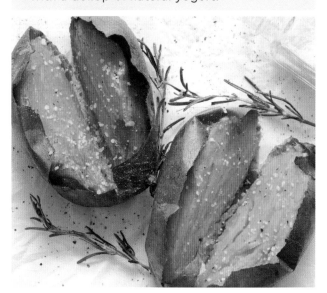

At dinner time, depending on how late I am and how heavy a meal I want, I either have soups (such as lentil or minestrone), stews or stir-fries – often with added protein. I try to make my own sauces – basically, anything I can make myself I do, rather than buying it in a packet. Just looking at the ingredients and levels of salt, sugar and additives in a packet sauce motivates me to create my own. You know what's going into it and you know that you're not adding any extra non-foods.

Once you're used to home cooking, I think that these dishes taste better. It's easy to get stuck in a pattern of buying packaged foods and extras and your tastebuds get used to it. Now I find most bought sauces too salty and sugary for me – I much prefer a cheaper homecooked alternative where possible.

Here's one of my simple stir-fry sauce recipes:

FAVOURITE STIR-FRY SAUCE
(SERVES 1–2)

Ingredients:
- 200ml (6¾fl oz) vegetable stock (homemade if possible)
- Juice of 1 lemon
- 1 tbsp sesame oil
- 2 tbsp light soy sauce
- 1–2 tsp cornflour/cornstarch

Method:
Mix together all the wet ingredients, then add the cornflour at the end to help thicken your sauce. Add to your stir fry for the last 4–5 minutes of the cooking time.

Eat More Veg

I'm vegetarian – I've also been vegan but I found that my body felt better with some dairy as well – and I love experimenting with seasonal vegetable dishes. I love gnocchi and use the recipe below, bringing in spinach for extra nutrition:

SPINACH GNOCCHI (SERVES 2)

Ingredients:

- 500g (1lb 2oz) floury potatoes
- 75g (2⅔oz) fresh spinach
- 2 medium egg yolks
- 125g (4½oz) plain/all-purpose flour

Method:

Cook the potatoes and mash. Wilt the spinach by pouring boiling water over it, leave for 2 minutes, then drain well. Squeeze all the liquid out of it and chop. Mix together the potatoes, spinach and egg yolks, then add the flour and mix well. Shape into small balls and chill for 30 minutes. Cook them in boiling water for about 4 minutes. This dish is so worth the effort. Try making a simple pesto as the sauce.

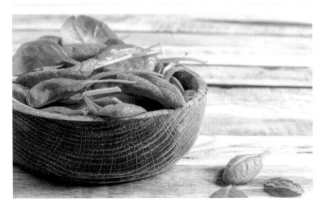

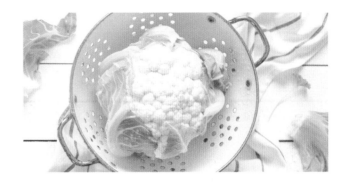

Cauliflower is another brilliant and versatile vegetable. I make cauliflower tacos – adding some soy sauce and honey onto the florets and roasting them, then piling them into a taco with shredded cabbage marinated in a white wine vinegar with a little honey. The flavours are so good! Or try my ...

STICKY CAULIFLOWER WITH BROWN RICE (SERVES 2–3)

Ingredients:

- 1 cauliflower, washed
- Dash of light soy sauce
- Dash of honey
- Squeeze of garlic paste
- 3 tbsp rice wine vinegar
- 1 tbsp cornflour/cornstarch
- 200g (6¾oz) long-grain brown rice, cooked and drained to serve

Method:

Cut the cauliflower into florets. Mix together the rest of the ingredients, except the rice, in a pan and heat until thickened. Pour the sauce over the cauliflower and bake at 200°C (400°F) for 50 minutes. Serve with brown rice.

Baking happens too. I enjoy making a cake – I just try not to add too much white sugar where possible. If I think the recipe doesn't need as much as it says, I'll try less or use a different type of sugar, such as coconut sugar, or sometimes apple puree instead. I look for ways to get that sweetness without refined sugar. I like experimenting, and most of the time my recipes turn out really well.

Try things – don't be afraid of using new foods and different combinations. Do anything to avoid getting things out of packets where possible. Many of my favourite meals are one-pot dishes and stews, which aren't fiddly or expensive – it's about packing the dishes with flavour so that your tastebuds get a lot of satisfaction. You can create so much with just a good recipe and basic ingredients.

Hydrate, Hydrate, Hydrate!

I was so bad at hydration growing up. Again, I didn't understand its importance until I was older. It helps with everything – your digestion, sleep, energy, concentration, skin and so much more. I was drinking all these pop drinks and thought that was fine. I didn't realize I needed even more water to cancel them out.

Now I restrict myself to a maximum of two caffeinated coffees a day – as I need my coffee – and I'll have a full glass of room-temperature water before my first coffee of the day. That sets me up after all night with nothing to drink.

I also have a water bottle with the hours of the day marked on it, so I can see how much I'm drinking – I don't always hit the target every day, but it does help me stay on top of my hydration.

Sometimes adding pieces of lemon, orange or lime to my water makes it more interesting. Then I drink a lot of green tea, which is also hydrating and good for you (though it does have a little caffeine in it).

I used to drink a lot more alcohol than I do now, and then I began to realize the effect it had on my body. The more fit I felt with my healthy eating habits, the more I could feel the effects of the alcohol and what it was doing to my body – I started to feel a lot more ill the day after drinking. I put that down to my body doing all the right things and feeling really good and then being hit with the alcohol and sugar that my body wasn't used to anymore.

Relish Everything in Moderation

The people in the Blue Zones, who are living healthier and longer lives, have diets full of fish and vegetables. However, they are still drinking wine, eating cheese and not restricting themselves anything. The key is that they are active, eat plenty of wholefoods and probably have plenty of communal meals together. To really "feed" your body, concentrate on eating more natural things and enjoying them. Find the joy in your food.

The perfect diet should not just keep you alive, it should let you thrive.

> "Try things – don't be afraid of using new foods and different combinations."

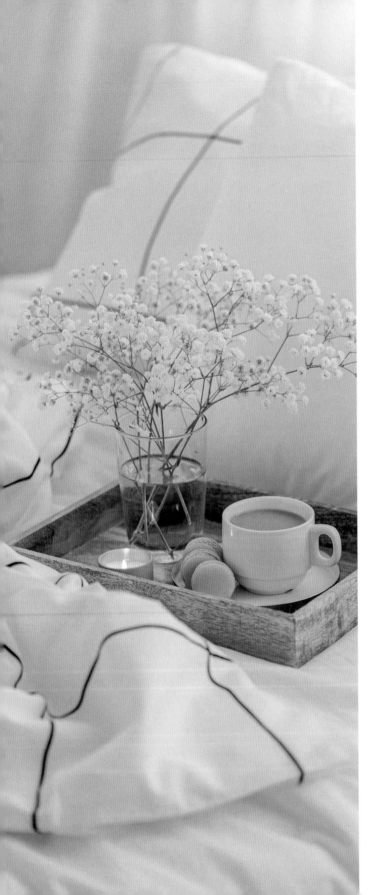

THE POWER OF REST

It might seem strange that, in a book focusing on exercise, I'm very keen to talk about rest and downtime and its importance to body and brain. Time out that is not just rest on the sofa while creating the shopping list or tapping out emails – proper spiritual, emotional and physical rest.

When I was younger, I felt that my body was invincible so I just kept going, but now I know that I need regular rest and downtime. On a day off, I don't worry about doing any more than I need to – I treat it as a rest day.

When I'm teaching someone, I reassure them too that their body has limits. Whether you're running a race, at the gym or dancing – you're using every muscle in your body, and also your brain, so you need to allow for rest to get the most out of the experience. If you keep pushing and pushing, which is what I used to do, it's not beneficial.

Growing up as a dancer, I was always trying to practise more and work harder for longer to be "the best". There was a sense that putting in the hours and making the sacrifices, left, right and centre was the only route to success. Other dancers would ask, "How many hours did you practise this week?" And instantly you would want to go big, to have put in more hours, as if that made you a better dancer. I thought I was invincible. I knew my body was getting tired, but I just didn't allow myself to acknowledge that, to the point that I had to stop dancing for months when I became ill. From that moment on, I knew that I had to find time to fit rest into my schedule. It became a priority in my life.

I think that many of us feel this way. Maybe you feel you need to be the last person in the office or the one doing the most hours in training, or maybe you take on extra jobs and say yes to everything. Modern life is busy – we are often taking on responsibility for others, working to get the next promotion or juggling various demands. We're told that this is "normal", that it's what is necessary to get where you want to be, to be "a success", to do what needs to be done, or to be happy.

Rest Shouldn't Make You Feel Guilty

I used to feel guilty about taking time off and again that was pressure in my head, which made me feel anxious and stressed and think I couldn't stop. I love being busy, busy, busy and having plans and goals and dreams, but it's easy to be consumed by everything in your life.

I had to learn how to take care of myself and how important rest and "switching off" are for mind and body, to power down and recover between periods of work. It felt counterintuitive that an intense training session followed by time to allow my mind to process things and my muscles to rest was actually more beneficial than being in the dance studio for eight or nine hours straight. Giving

yourself that time to rest and to allow your brain to switch off, as well as moving more, is at the heart of this whole book.

And it's something you need to constantly monitor. For example, in the first Covid lockdown, I tried to do so much. Instead of pacing my work and plans, and getting so much more out of what I was trying to achieve, I filled my schedule every single day then I crashed and ended up doing nothing for a while – it was frustrating!

Do You Schedule Rest?

We don't put downtime in our diaries – we fill up our days and weekends with back-to-back activities and work and "fun things" that we need to do or should do, but we rarely ever schedule an hour to do nothing, to simply concentrate on nourishing ourselves. We're all guilty of eating lunch at our desks or on the job often. What does this say about our priorities in life? In the nine hours between breakfast and dinner, how much time are you allowing yourself to switch off from work or your other responsibilities? And how do you feel about that time? Are you snatching a break to watch a quick burst of TV or doom-scrolling on your phone?

It's crucial to force yourself to look for the space you need – in your day, your week and your year. I never used to do this but it's something I now consciously practice. Ideally, booking in half a day a month to "reset" is a great idea if you can find the time. That time will pay itself back many times over in your increased happiness and focus. At the other end of the scale, even something as simple as taking three minutes a day to just sit still and relax your mind and your body is a start. Think of ways you can increase the rest in your daily life.

Sleep it Off

Of course, as well as taking a break, sleep is so important. When we're busy and trying to juggle things, sleep can be the first thing to suffer. Working late, waking in the night or not being able to relax into a deep sleep really affects the brain and the systems of the body. Consistent quality sleep and hitting your seven to eight hours a night is crucial.

I tend to be an early riser – sorry! It's just a natural thing for me. I don't like to set an alarm and I just wake up early and am awake straight away. I'll have my walk around the garden and get some fresh air and light, which is said to be very good for our bodies' natural (circadian) rhythms, helping us to sleep better. Without my seven to eight hours, I feel rubbish and like I can't tackle the world as I normally would. I'm a worrier at heart, so a lack of sleep can make my concerns feel much bigger than they really are.

In the evening, unless I'm back from work late, I like to have my dinner early-ish so my body feels replenished. I might watch a favourite programme on TV, then I often go to bed quite early. I make my bedroom a comfort zone. I might light a candle while I get ready for bed or listen to some ASMR (autonomous sensory meridian response) sounds to relax me. I make an effort not to go into the bedroom during the day too much – unless I take five minutes at some point for a restful break. I keep the bedroom as my sleeping space, so I look forward to going to that room at night. If I go there too much in the day, or let my work or hobby paraphernalia or papers take over the space, then I feel as if I should be doing something when I'm in there. Keeping the room as my sleeping space is a signal to my brain that it is now time to sleep.

Think about ways to streamline your sleeping area, and your night-time routine in order to send yourself a strong signal about the importance of sleep and shutting off.

Finding Sanctuary

My bedroom is where I go to relax and sleep, but I created another space upstairs in my home that is my haven. I feel completely calm in that place – it puts a smile on my face when I walk in. It's like a little hug room that makes me feel very safe and secure. Why not create something similar for yourself? It doesn't need to be a big space, just a little corner that you can make your own. I have flowers in the room, which make me feel special, and candles – I want it to communicate relaxation via all of my senses. And it makes me feel free to do whatever I want in that space. Sometimes I do my yoga there, but if I don't feel like yoga, I just go and sit in there. I might also get crafty some days and I enjoy painting. I put some music on and listen to that and craft or paint.

Creativity

I try to make time to do something different from whatever project I'm currently involved with – a not-so-obvious way of taking a break. It's good to

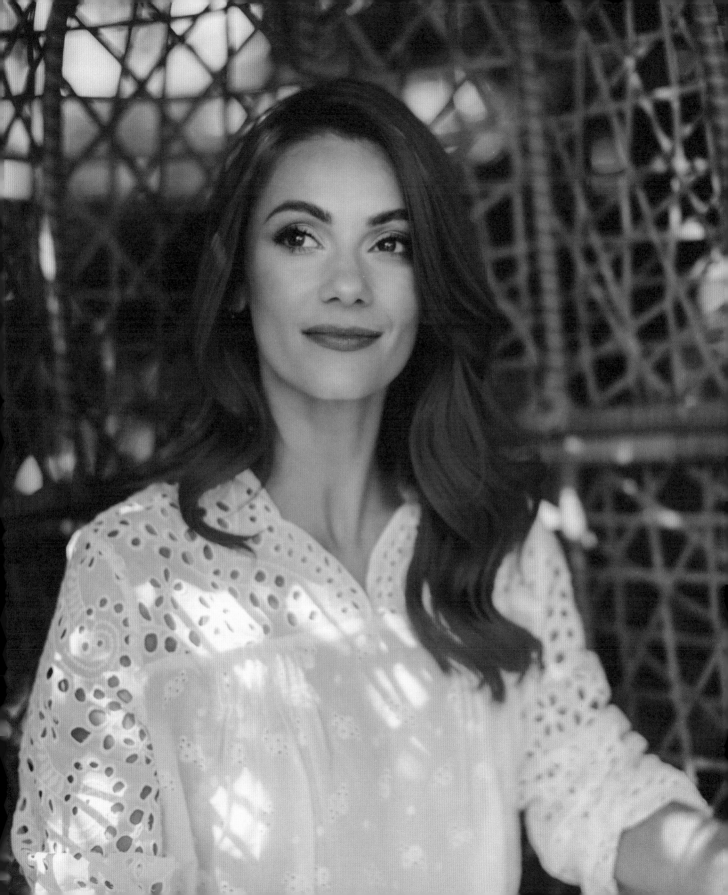

try something different and to feel like I'm doing something other than my job. Even when I love my job, I love it even more when I have a day off from it. I come back refreshed and I'm like, "Oh it's so good to be back!"

Trying something different in your free time is a great way to "rest" from your everyday stresses. I find creativity freeing – I get this through my dance and choreography, but I also love the idea of making things. Just something small, like a birthday card. It's a great feeling doing something for someone else, making them feel special.

I love writing letters to my mum and dad because I know that they enjoy receiving them and it also keeps me connected to home. And I write to my grandfather, Pop, who's about 95. I'll sit there in my little space to write – I get so much from finding that time to connect with people I love and to show people that I'm thinking of them. My life is so unpredictable with how much I tour that keeping in touch with family and friends from all over the world is difficult. Again, it might sound forced, but making a conscious effort to connect with loved ones is something I make an effort to do, otherwise I know that my work schedule would take over.

Boundaries and Saying "No"

We all feel that pressure to perform, to always be "on", to show up and say "yes". It's certainly rife in the entertainment industry. There can be a lot of pressure to work harder than anyone else, to tick everything off the to-do list or make everyone happy.

It's incredibly empowering to be able to say a graceful "no". It is a very powerful word and everyone should use it more often! We must actively choose what we're going to do and do it well. Focus your time and energy on what you can fit into your week and enjoy it, rather than doing far more activities but getting stressed racing from one venue to another.

We've all been out to celebrate someone's birthday after a crazy week at work when we know we need to be at home in bed. We show up because we feel we have to, because it seems easier than making the tough decision, or explaining to someone how you need a break for yourself. We've all wasted hours of our precious time doing things because we "should" do them or we said "yes" without allowing ourselves time to properly consider what we already had on our plate. The big truth is that it's absolutely fine to say, "I'm not going to fit that in" or "I'd love to but it's not something I have the capacity for this week" or "Could we take a raincheck until next month when I've got more money?" It's not a failure to say no, to turn down an invitation, to *not* have the time to support a friend's fundraising event ... It's about taking control of your energy and your time. Two precious things we give away so readily to things that aren't necessarily priorities in our lives. Be honest and realistic about what you can achieve in your waking hours.

What are you saying "yes" to that means you have to say "no" to something else? What's disappearing from your week when you say "yes" to something? Extra time at work might be a positive if you're working toward a promotion or finishing a major project, or it could also be a negative habit that you've got into that is impacting on your self-care time. What things in the past weeks could you have said "no" to but didn't, and why?

There have been a lot of wonderful events and opportunities that I've turned down, especially in the last few years, because I've just gone "I don't have time (but I want to)." If I say "yes" to all these things, I know I'm not going to have time to rest, or to see family or friends or take time for myself. Spending time with those closest to me is another rest and relaxation thing – it boosts my mood. I know it's super important to schedule in time for those things – I need them in my life.

Breathe Your Way to Calm

Just as clearing your bedroom or creating a sanctuary space are ways to encourage more rest, there are tools we can use to send our bodies a clear message to take a break. Sometimes when I've been dancing in shows, I find it hard to wind down afterwards – just as many people find it hard to calm down after a busy, tough day. When this happens, my go-to wind-down superpower is my breath. It's so simple, yet so effective in calming the body. It works by sending the body a clear message to switch off the fight-or-flight response that stress and life often invokes. Like meditation and yoga, changing your breathing helps you to slow down, relax and become calm. Your heart rate drops, your blood pressure lowers and more oxygen floods your body.

Long exhalations are helpful for me – for example, if I'm about to dance on *Strictly* and I'm feeling a little nervous, instead of focusing on the breath in (which can make you feel a little more panicky), I focus on the breath out. I take a normal breath in and try to take a long breath out, which seems to sort of slow everything down a little. When I'm feeling nervous, that helps dramatically. Here are some favourite techniques:

THE 4–7–8 TECHNIQUE (BY ANDREW WEIL)

I find this technique helpful if I'm in bed and feeling very awake. When I get like this – tired but busy in my head and thinking "Why am I not sleeping?" – I find this calms me and helps me have a better night of sleep. It also works if I wake up in the middle of the night.

- Get comfortable in a seated or lying position and take 3 or 4 deep, slow breaths.
- Then, breathe in slowly for a count of 4.
- Hold the breath for a count of 7, then make a long exhale for a count of 8. Repeat for 4 rounds.

It may feel forced at first, but take your time to find your rhythm and relax into the breathing and you will feel the difference.

ALTERNATE NOSTRIL BREATHING

If I'm on my own, and feeling stressed, I use alternate nostril breathing – simply sealing one nostril with a finger or thumb and breathing normally, then doing the same on the other side. It feels good if I have more time and can do it for ten minutes or so.

- Get yourself comfortable in a seated or lying position and take 3 or 4 deep, slow breaths.
- Then, breathe in slowly through your left nostril, holding your right nostril closed with your right thumb, pause briefly at the top of the breath, then breathe out through the right nostril, holding the left nostril shut with the ring finger of your right hand.
- Then, breathe in through your right nostril, pause at the top of the breath and switch so you are holding your right nostril closed with your right thumb. Breathe out through your left nostril. Repeat for 5 minutes.

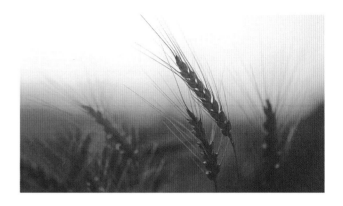

LION'S BREATH

A particular favourite of mine is Lion's Breath, to relieve stress and tension in mind and upper body. There's something so releasing about making a noise when you breathe out, and it just makes you feel in tune with your body. It's probably more of a thing to do on your own, as it can be a little awkward to do when in a room with others!

- Start with 3 or 4 deep, slow breaths.
- Then, on the next exhale, open your mouth wide, stick out your tongue, pointing it down toward your chin and exhale forcefully with a "ha" sound.
- Continue breathing normally for about 5 breaths, then repeat the roar. Repeat 6 times.

I learned to use my breathing to make me feel calmer and stronger through yoga, and I use these techniques frequently.

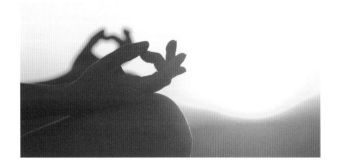

Meditation

I have to own up that I used to see meditation as a bit of a fad. I thought "Who's got time for that?" I tried it once and thought, "Oh, that didn't work." It wasn't until I decided to give it a proper try that I came to realize its power. And it takes a while. It's not something that makes this big difference straight away, especially if you're a busy person and have a lot on your mind. You have to practise – I kept trying and trying and trying until I went, "Ah, that's what it does. I understand it now."

It doesn't mean you have to sit there for hours feeling all full of peace and love either. Our brains are always on, our phones are always with us and we're always connected in some way to work and stress, so just by putting your phone away and trying to distance yourself from the constant mania in your head is a start. I like to use something to focus on in my meditation, such as listening to one particular sound. We don't really do this in everyday life – just focus on one thing in the present without having to react, or process it, or do something about it. It's refreshing to allow ourselves that space, and it can be done anywhere or anytime – on a train or the bus, when you're stirring dinner or on a run. It takes your brain away from all the mental chatter. Though if you want to use a calm space at home for your mindfulness, that's great too.

I find that being mindful in small chunks of time helps me to refocus and clear my mind when I need that brain break. I often use an app, such as Calm, or find a simple routine on YouTube to follow.

I also enjoy ASMR (autonomous sensory meridian response), which is another way into mindfulness as a relaxation tool. Again, it uses mainly sound to relax the body and quieten the mind. I could listen to it for hours.

Time Out

I have a very strong work ethic, which I got from my parents. When I was growing up, my mum and dad were always working. I never saw them stop and have a break. In fact, if we ever stopped and sat and watched TV as a kid, my mum would ask "Why are you not doing something or cleaning your room?" I would have sneak into the lounge to watch TV when they weren't around! It meant that I always have this need to be doing something set in my mentality, and to change that vibe takes constant effort for me.

Realizing that rest is as important as being active helped me begin to make proper decisions about how I spent my time and what really mattered to me. Putting my physical health first also meant I was valuing my mental health more. Setting myself realistic goals and saying "no" have helped me to become comfortable with taking time out.

This mindset is about feeling OK about taking an hour or the day off, or to let your body do its own thing. The truth is that you're better off doing one set of really good squats than rushing through a thousand squats the wrong way, fitting one activity into your afternoon rather than three, and not trying to outperform your way through life. Take your time to work properly on your choices ... and then rest.

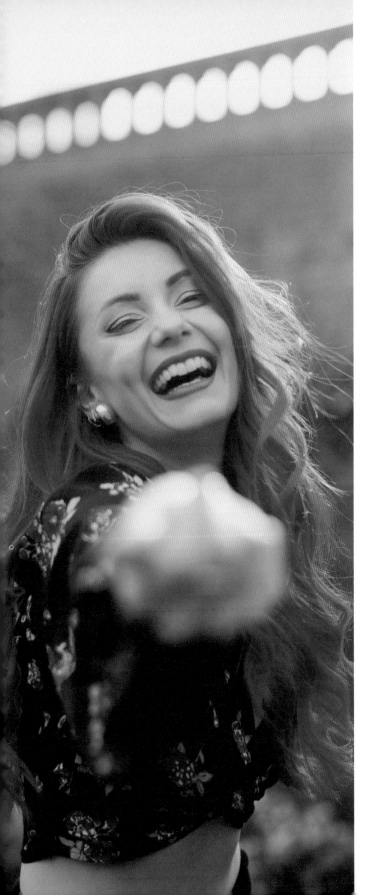

THE POWER OF POSITIVITY

The final of the Four Pillars is positivity. I've spoken a lot about joy and finding joy in how we live. I think it's important to recognize that finding happiness often takes purposeful action from us – to focus on what is important to us, and to make time in our lives to prioritize that. When was the last time you put aside your responsibilities and pressures and did something purely for yourself? Just because you wanted to and without thoughts of anyone else? How easy do you find it to rise above worries and stresses, or what others think or expect of you?

It's easy to get into the habit of feeling guilt and negativity about doing stuff for ourselves, but it's not selfish at all to put yourself first and make your own needs and happiness a priority. I don't care if I spend all day doing things for myself. It doesn't make me feel selfish, it makes me happy and grounded, and stronger and healthier. I smile more and stand taller when I'm making time for myself. And that makes those around me happy as well.

Be Positive

People tell me that I'm always cheerful and upbeat about things, that I don't seem to let things get to me, but the reality is that, like most of us, I struggle sometimes to stay positive and keep going during the tough times.

Worry is one of the things I do. I get a bit anxious at times, and it stops me from doing things. If I worry about something, I procrastinate and I struggle to get anything done. Simply being kinder to ourselves makes a huge difference, reassuring ourselves and not pressuring ourselves is so important – and, importantly, within our own control.

For example, when I'm going to dance live, rather than worry whether the crowd are going to like it or not, I reassure myself that the crowd are going to love it and stand up and clap at the end. If you're reassuring yourself that they're out there enjoying themselves rather than putting pressure on yourself thinking "I really hope that they like this", it's automatically easier to deal with. Reassurance rather than pressure.

Three phrases that I use to ease my worries have really helped me:

#1 "IT'S NOT MY BUSINESS WHAT THEY'RE THINKING!"

It's natural to worry what are people are going to think if you wear this/do this/say that. When I find that niggling in my head, I tell myself it's not my business what someone else thinks. It's none of my business what someone else thinks of my outfit, laugh or funny story – they can think whatever they want, and they will. This is such a good way to remind yourself that other people's reactions to what you do are about *them* – *their* thoughts, *their* choices, *their* experiences. It makes it easier to bring your thoughts back to what you want, and not let the reactions of others dictate your choices.

#2 "I'M NOT THAT IMPORTANT!"

What? It's true though. I'm important to myself, to my family and friends, but to most other people, I'm not. Most people are busy worrying about their own lives – they don't have time to worry about others. If someone says something about you, you think that they're thinking that 24/7. But no. You're not that important to them. They might think something about you for a split second, but the rest of the time they're actually thinking about what they're having for breakfast, or their own problems. In your head, you build it up – but you're really not that important to 99% of the people you meet.

This might not a nice thing to hear – but it's an effective way to put your worries into perspective.

#3 "WILL I REMEMBER THIS IN A YEAR'S TIME?"

Think back over the past five years – can you remember a bunch of times that really worried you – maybe a party you didn't want to go to because you knew you wouldn't know anyone there, or a presentation you had to give at work or college? You'll probably have to think really hard to remember these incidents because they're in the past and, guess what, you got through the worry and the stress and came out the other side. Many things in life are stressful while they're happening, but if you can appreciate that it's not a life-changing scenario and that it will soon be over and done with, it can really dampen your worrying thoughts.

Social Media

I'm so glad that social media wasn't around when I was young. The peer pressure and the effects of social media are an immense factor in how we feel day today – often without us even realizing.

It was a real shock when my social media grew. I'd always had a lot of positive people on my social – just a few hundred people I knew and friends. Then, all of a sudden, people I didn't know started to follow me. I struggled with it for a while – and still do now sometimes – and I had to decide how to deal with that.

Social media can be a force for good in many ways, but it can be bad too. For example, I got a message recently saying that I had really let myself go and wasn't looking that great anymore. While I decided in the past to only read messages from people that I know and to block trolls immediately, sometimes it's hard not to look. Things like that – you tell yourself that you won't let it bother you, and it's not anyone that you know. But it plays on your mind. I thought about that comment more than once. I did the "It's not my business what they're thinking" line, but this is something that I shouldn't have to deal with. It's hard knowing the messages are there, even if I do choose to ignore them, but I try not to let this take up my headspace.

Journaling and Talking

I talk to a therapist about how I am feeling if I'm struggling with something. Having someone to talk to is a great tool if you're feeling anxious. I realize that not everyone can get a therapist, but even writing down your feelings is hugely therapeutic. Journaling or writing gives you the time and space to admit and understand your concerns and explore where they're coming from. I'm someone who can struggle to talk about things out loud, but writing it down and reading it back later helps me to identify what I'm really thinking. Even going into a room by yourself and saying – or shouting – things out loud so that the fear is not in your body and causing tension helps to release it. Whether verbally or on paper, sharing your worry, putting it into words and exploring why you feel this way is fundamental to taking control of your emotions and removing the power from your fears.

Affirmations

Affirmation cards are another effective tool to nurture good mental health – uplifting tokens that I write or select in the morning for the day ahead. The thoughts we direct our mind toward have power. I keep the cards where I can see them during the day, and they give me a boost – just reading a simple and positive quote, or a compliment from someone, gives encouragement. And we all need that sometimes.

My Circle of Life

It's all very well talking about "making time for ourselves" and self-care, as well as eating well and moving more, but for many of us that's just talk. Finding time to put ourselves first or take rest time is tricky unless we forge ways to make it happen. There is a great tool I use to look at my week and help me to make tough but good decisions about what I'm doing.

I draw a "Wheel of Life" for the week ahead and use it to understand how I'm spending my time. I literally just draw a circle on a piece of paper and divide it into pie slices to represent the key areas of my life, the important things I want to spend my time on. I might divide my week into:

- Free time/rest time/self-care time
- Friends and family/relationship with partner
- Career/work
- Movement/exercise
- Creativity/activities
- Sleep

Choose the priorities you have in your life at this time. Maybe focus on your current concerns or aims; add in "cooking good food" or "reading" if these are things you want to aim to find extra time for. You are in control of how your time is represented.

Next I look at my diary for the week and see what I have on. Some weeks are crazier than others, but generally my work will be in there, and perhaps some time seeing friends. But I can look at the rest of my time and check when some downtime can be found. I look for times when I can grab an hour or two to relax or do a yoga class, or catch up on a creative project.

Then I look at these different aspects of my life and ask myself: What are the issues with my time? What am I missing this week? Then I build a plan of action to find more time for what is important to me, to strike a balance.

It makes me feel so much better to just make it clearer in my mind, to have this tool to view how my life is dividing up. Everyone will use it differently. I like to make mine on a Monday morning, but you could do it at the end of the week, or a couple of times each week. Once I've drawn it, I write up a plan of action for myself. If I'm feeling that the "friends" aspect of my life is missing and I haven't connected with important people, I write a note in my diary for a time to phone a couple of friends sometime in the week. Thinking about and making a plan for these tiny little things allows me to set the intention to make them happen.

Vision Board for Focus

Banishing worries and clarifying your priorities for the week helps clear the way to more proactive thought patterns, rather than being reactive to what is going on around you. Taking control of my thoughts and planning my time is key to my mental strength and focus. I have been lucky – being involved in a competitive sport from an early age helped me to set goals and understand how it was necessary to identify what I was trying to achieve, and to work at getting to that place. Of course I didn't always get what I wanted, but I have my own ways to keep clear in my mind what is important to me – in the short- and long-term. Goals are important – as long as you have reasonable goals that recognize your capacity and time, and you've given yourself enough time to realize them.

I create a vision board regularly. This is a visual representation of my future goals – I like to see what I'm aiming for. Using the power of visualization, you put together a collage of images and words that represent your short- and long-term aims. Why not take an afternoon to find inspiration in magazines or online and build your board using cardboard, corkboard or whatever you have to hand? Once you've made it, put it somewhere you will look at it regularly, such as above your desk or next to a mirror. You could even make it your screensaver.

It's not about putting pressure on yourself, rather it's to clarify your aims and make a reminder and prompt for those goals. I use a board each year to focus on the things I want to achieve in the next 12 months. It could be anything from a special holiday in a particular place to focusing on my health or moving house. I look at the images frequently and visualize my life when I have reached the goals, thinking about how achieving those goals is going to make me feel – it's a great meditation.

The key to making this tool a success is not to put your board up, sit back and wait for your dreams to come true. It's not that simple. The vision board supports you to focus on your dreams. To make them come true you must have a clear indication of how you are going to achieve them. Break down your aims into clear steps and actions. Writing them down is a great way to hold yourself accountable. For example, noting down what you

want, the steps to achieve this and what you need to do to action your plan.

Breaking down aims into small steps makes big change possible in ways that fit into our life, to introduce new habits and build new routines. Understanding what motivates and is important to you is the first step toward lasting change.

Self-Care Day

Finally, one of my favourite ways to get back on track after a stressful period or when I'm feeling low on mental resilience – and to recommend to others when I see them feeling off-colour – is a self-care day. It feels amazing! It's easy to "allow" yourself half an hour here and there for some R&R, but the reality is that me-time tends to be bottom of the list. There's always a last-minute trip to the post office you forgot was necessary, or a phone call from a friend you've been meaning to speak to for ages …. Taking a complete day for yourself makes you set boundaries firmly – and gives you proper space to relax. Why not schedule something creative or some pampering, or arrange to see people? Taking a day means that I have time to relax into me-time and have some distance from work and everyday admin to fully relax and see the bigger picture of how life is going at the time and if I'm on track with where I want to be. It's a day when I can set myself some goals for the coming months.

I have always loved the feeling of being pampered, so a self-care day for me may involve getting my hair done. I remember going to the hairdresser when I was young, of sitting there and someone touching my hair. And they'd ask my mum "Does she need a shampoo?" And I'd say "Yes – please!" For me, there were always two things in life I wanted to do – dancing and hairdressing. I'm not sure where my love of hairdressing came from. I grew up playing with Barbie dolls and I would colour their hair with food colouring or give them interesting cuts. When I was about eight, I performed my first "real" haircut on my dad with kitchen scissors, which went surprisingly well!

It's the creativity that appealed to me – and making someone else feel special. I trained for four years and then opened my own salon before I took up dancing professionally. People would come to the salon, and they genuinely loved getting their hair done because they knew that when they left, they were going to feel good about themselves. And you can say, "I made that happen, I created that."

Doing something special for yourself is the most fun way to send a message of positivity to your brain, to put a smile on your face and to remind yourself to cherish yourself, body and mind.

> "Taking a day means that I have time to relax into me-time and have some distance from work and everyday admin to fully relax and see the bigger picture of how life is going at the time and if I'm on track with where I want to be."

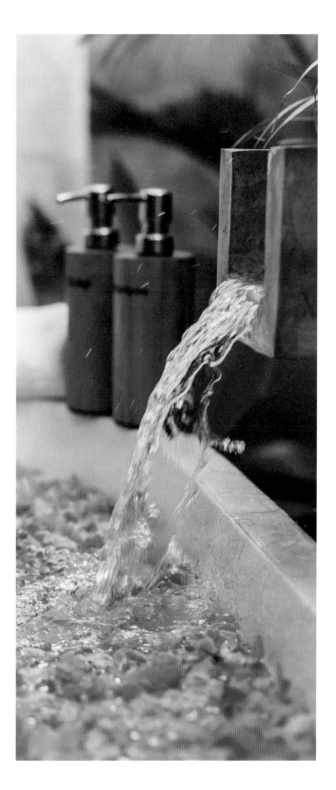

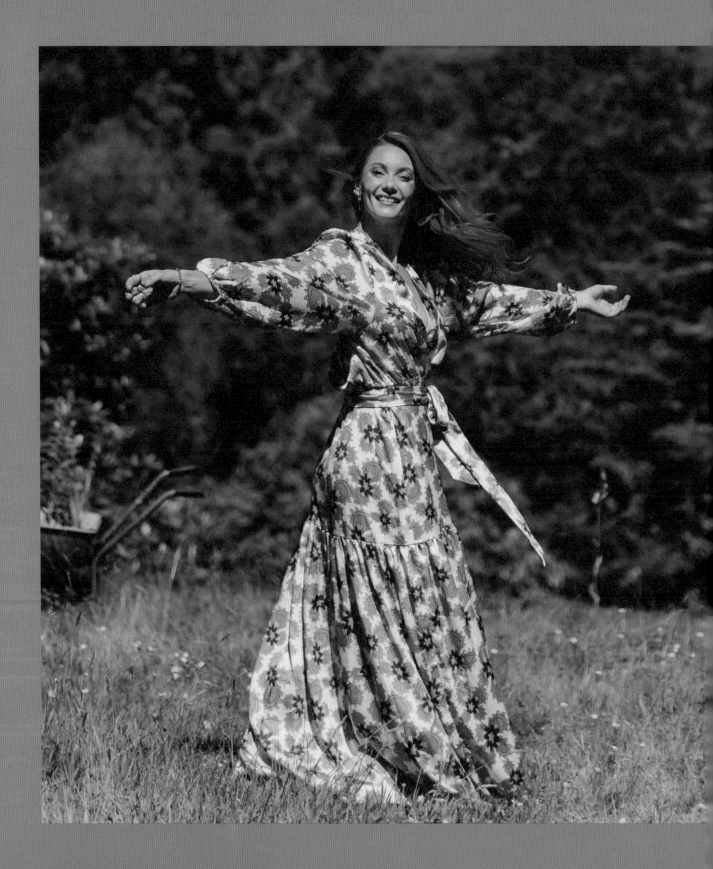

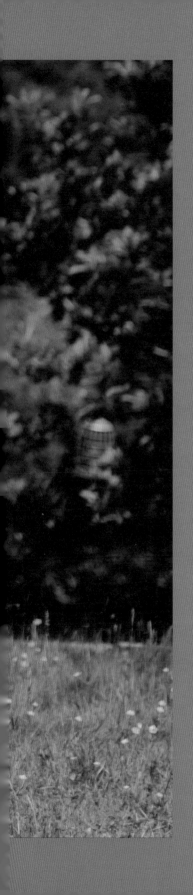

Part 2

The

Movements

Are you ready to get moving? To help kick off your new relationship with exercise I'm going to show you how to do a range of my favourite dance, Pilates and yoga moves. In Part 3 of the book, I'll bring these moves together in 21 energizing, fun and quick workout routines as part of my **21 Days to a Stronger, Happier You** plan. But first, let's explore each of the three forms of movement in turn – first dance, then Pilates, then yoga – each time getting to grips with my handpicked selection of moves in a step-by-step way – so that you can see for yourself why they are such great ways to enjoy movement, making you feel better in both body and mind.

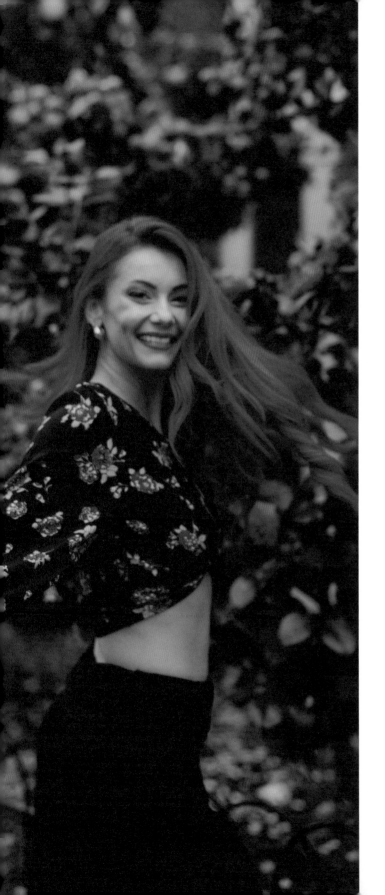

DANCE MOVES TO TONE AND ENERGIZE

Most people associate me with dance – they think that's my main exercise (and some of the time it is). It can intimidate people when they know that I have so many years of dance experience and training – friends don't tend to ask me if I want to hit the dance floor much!

Beyond the hours of competitive dance, training and rehearsals though, dance is personal to each and every one of us. Maybe you have no problems throwing some shapes at a kitchen disco or busting moves when your favourite song calls to you – but for many of us, dancing is something that we only do at a party or event. We might love watching it, but it's not something we consider part of our daily life.

I'd love dance to be something that everyone does every day – that we think about as a form of movement that we should be doing at least five times a week. It's joyful and empowering – and probably the one form of exercise that everyone can do (even if they don't think they can!) – and that makes you smile. There's no training or equipment required, you can do it any time you want to, on your own or out with friends, and to practically every and any kind of music – or none at all. There is no right or wrong way to dance, no "shoulds" or restrictions. It's simply about the enjoyment of moving your body.

I also love the theatre of dance – the way it allows you to express yourself in your own unique way. There's a reason why we dance at special occasions – to show love, happiness, to attract a mate, to release tension, to be creative or to have pure fun. Dancing elevates our mood and boosts our endorphins – and the fact that it's about moving our body in so many healthy ways is an added bonus.

When we talk about the power of movement to unite body and mind, and to lift our mood, surely we are talking first and foremost about dance.

Letting Go

I started dance as a child, and that perhaps explains my natural passion for dancing and for finding enjoyment in the way I move my body. When we're young, our inhibitions and awareness of what society dictates we "should" do are at their weakest, so dance and movement come to us easily and freely. As children, we didn't walk – we ran, skipped, hopped, jumped or crawled. Children are happiest sprawling on the floor, bouncing at all angles on trampolines and swinging on monkey bars. Movement in all directions is easy and fun; sitting still is quite tricky. And if you watch children moving around or dancing, their posture and movement looks so natural and healthy. So when and why do so many of us stop dancing for fun?

Learning so many forms of dance – and I'm still learning new moves and styles – is a huge honour.

And now I find that introducing others to dance via teaching means a lot to me, too! It gives me just so much pleasure to be able to pass on my dancing knowledge and skills, but what is most powerful is the way I can show people how much fun comes with movement, and how we connect more deeply with our bodies through dance. That's what I often see in the people I've taught – the newfound sense of fun and connection! Even if they don't carry on dancing for hours each week, I know that they have found their sweet spot in their relationship with movement and that they've discovered how good regular exercise makes them feel, with its huge benefits for both mood and energy. It becomes an essential in their lives.

Different Grooves

Choosing what dance styles and moves to include in this book was tricky. Different styles help me understand the mechanics of the body in different ways and suit different moods on different days.

Firstly, I've included eight moves from ballet, which is the ultimate form of body conditioning. Perhaps you've tried something similar with a barre class? I was late to the ballet scene but soon realized what it could bring to my ballroom and Latin dancing. I started ballet when I was about 15, so I had an immediate respect for it as it was so difficult to learn at that stage. I wished I'd done it when I was much younger.

Ballet was important for me in terms of learning a proper discipline in my movements, and it changed my posture and increased my awareness of the body. Latin is a very *freeing* dance style, and relies a lot on personality and performance – and I had that in buckets! But I found that strength, precision and the technicalities of ballet were more difficult for me. The sheer athleticism and stamina of the ballet dancers I have met is astounding, and the strictness of the movement work they do really sculpts their bodies. Ballet made me fully conscious of the alignment in my body as I dance, vastly improving my posture and my core strength, and helping me to understand what each of my muscles is doing. I also find it calming and soothing, easy to get into and so worthwhile in terms of how it makes my body feel – so it was an obvious choice to include here.

While ballet moves are about lengthening, strengthening and toning muscles (like Pilates in many ways), I also wanted to include some faster dances and Latin drama to encourage you to let yourself go and not worry about technique. Salsa was therefore an obvious choice for me to include – so I hope that my four key salsa moves get you shaking your hips as you burn up the floor. There's a reason that Zumba is a popular exercise class – the sizzling non-stop salsa moves that it involves boost endorphins, get your heart working and tone you up everywhere. Salsa is a high-energy dance with moves that will get your whole body swivelling to the Latin rhythms.

The fastest of the Latin dances is the jive, full of swinging moves and leg flicks. I chose four key moves from this dance, which stems from the 1930s and 40s, as they are relatively easy to pick up and, like salsa, can be done, if desired, in a way that is more about energy and fun than tricky technique.

I want you to jive away your cares with the hip-swinging action that these moves entail!

Finally, I chose three tap moves because there's something immensely uplifting about tip-tapping to the beat. Few can watch Fred Astaire or Gene Kelly and not want to pull on a pair of tap shoes and give it a go. The rhythm is what makes tap so addictive – I love the way that it creates its own beat, with the steps being so wonderfully musical! So, when you get to the tap section, put on some "tappy" shoes and find a wooden or tiled floor if possible, and you'll soon be stomping and shuffling across your space with style and panache! Feel free to grab your top hat and cane too, of course!

Our Bodies are All Different

I always tell people I dance with and teach that they should watch and enjoy other dancers but not compare themselves to anyone else. Whether you're 55 or 25, with or without dance experience, it doesn't matter – everyone I work with starts from a different place. Remember you're going up the ladder for yourself and no one else.

Each of us has a different body shape and physical strengths and weaknesses, and we all have our own relationship with dance and movement. It's really about making it enjoyable and doing it for yourself, not thinking "I have to do it like this" or "I should do what they do." In dance, your way of doing the moves is good – this is important to remember for all forms of exercise and working out. Do what your body will allow and what it needs.

Whether it's dance, yoga or Pilates, there will always be moves that you struggle with, depending

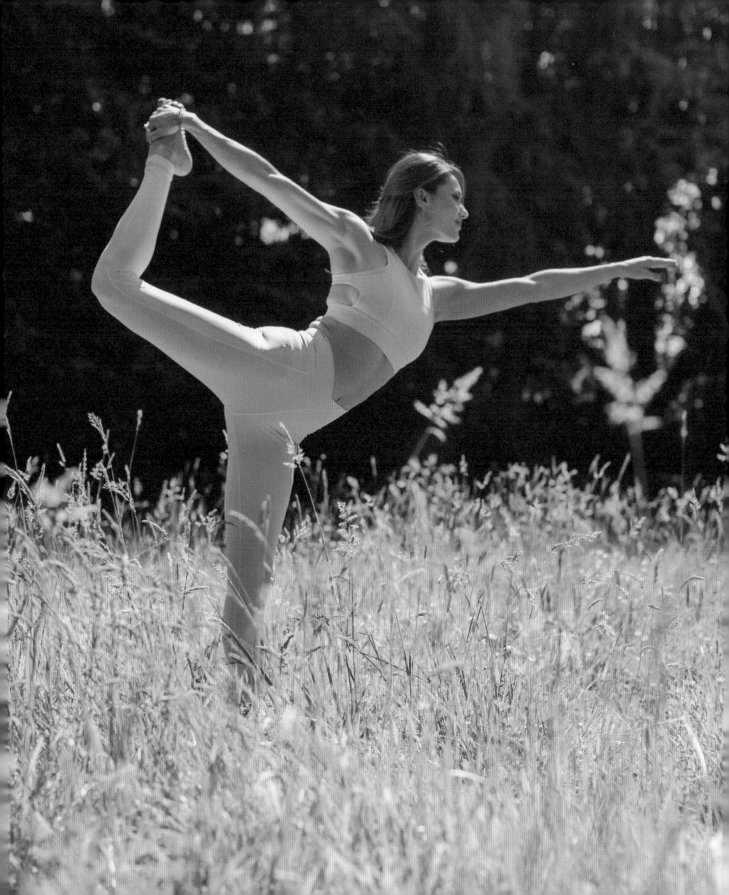

on the strengths and particularities of your body. There are moves and poses that I can't do – I just adjust them to make them achievable in my own way and I don't worry about it. I tell myself "my body can't do that, but I'll try it like this instead." My weakness is that I don't have open hips – mine are super tight and always have been. That's just the shape of my body. When I'm in a dance class and doing stretches, I might be told to do a butterfly stretch (to sit upright on the floor with feet touching and knees splayed to each side) and to get my knees close to the floor, but mine are still up by my ears! When I was younger that would bother me, but now I appreciate the strengths I have. For example, I have strong glutes (buttock muscles) and can comfortably stand on one leg, whereas some dancers with open hips might struggle with this.

So focus on what you can do and – as I always tell my students – show that off. It doesn't matter that my turnout is terrible and I'm not the most flexible dancer – that just shows that you don't have to be great in all areas to be a successful professional dancer. Everyone up there performing on a stage has something that they're not as good at, but you would never know as they focus on what they can do – on the positives. Any negative stuff about your wonderful body shouldn't take up any space in your head – it's best to move on from that.

Movement Shouldn't be Stressful

I hope you enjoy learning these new dance moves. If you find them difficult at first, or maybe finding and keeping the beat of your chosen music is foxing you, don't worry about it – keep going and keep smiling! When I'm teaching a routine to others and they're struggling, I have a secret tool to help them get over the hump. I might use this secret on "Terrible Tuesday" – when the routine is learned but not yet coming together properly; instead, it feels as if it's getting tougher as we finesse the technique and push ourselves really hard. In such instances, I'll stop and ask my partner what their favourite song is and tell them to forget everything I've told them about the technique and the routine, and just to move however they want for pure enjoyment. I'll put on a brilliant song – Miley Cyrus' "Party In The USA" is my all-time favourite for this – and watch them move with joy. Then I tell them to remember how it *feels* when they do this – as this is the feeling that dance should *always* give you. Even when

> Listen to my Spotify playlists to help you get in the mood to move! Search for:
>
> Move Yourself Happy – Dance
>
> Move Yourself Happy – Yoga & Pilates

you learn, or do, just one dance step, you want that feeling to still be there. So put that feeling into your movement for whatever time you have available to exercise each day – get the music on and just let go.

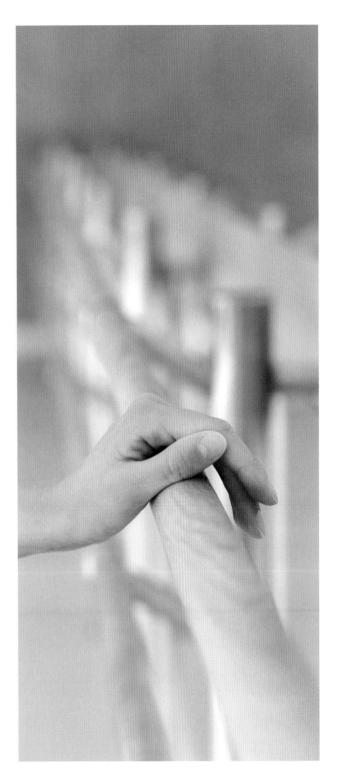

DANCE MOVES

1. BALLET – Arm Circles, Serving Food, Criss Cross, Up and Down
2. BALLET – Calf Raises
3. BALLET – Plié Squat
4. BALLET – Plié Squat with "Serving Food" Arms
5. BALLET – First to Second Position Squat Jump
6. BALLET – Curtsy Squat
7. BALLET – Lying Spine Twist
8. BALLET – Standing Leg Lifts
9. SALSA – Basic Step
10. SALSA – Basic Side-Step
11. SALSA – Zulu
12. SALSA – Spot Turn
13. JIVE – Forward and Side Kicks
14. JIVE – Chassé
15. JIVE – Toe Heel Step
16. JIVE – Jump Back with Clap
17. TAP – Ball Heel
18. TAP – Shuffle Tap
19. TAP – Shuffle Ball Heel

BALLET – ARM MOVEMENTS

Let's start with some simple ballet movements to tone up the arm muscles. All four of these moves should be done standing with the feet together.

ARM CIRCLES

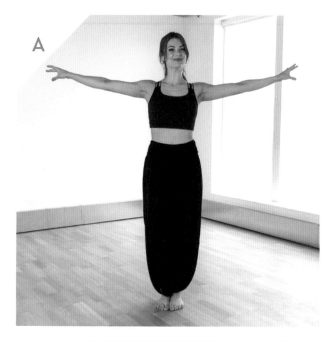

- Stand tall, extend your arms out to the sides at shoulder height, palms downward, and draw small circles with your arms, moving them both in the same direction. Start with small circles, then make them larger and larger, doing as many as you can in 60 seconds. **(A) (B)**
- Then do the same number of increasingly large circles in the other direction.
- To finish, slowly lower both arms.

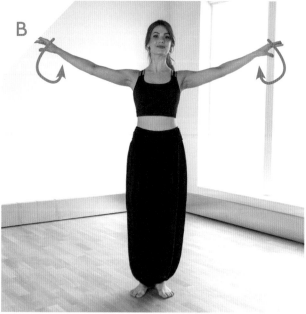

SERVING FOOD

- Stand tall, extend your arms out to the sides at shoulder height, with your palms upward. Then bring your arms to the front, keeping your palms upward, as if you were offering up a bowl of food. (A) (B)
- Bring your arms back out to the sides at shoulder height, then move them forward and backward as many times as you can in 60 seconds.
- To finish, lower your arms, twisting the palms down.

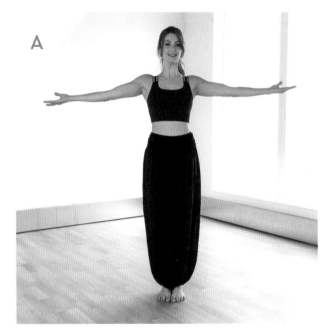

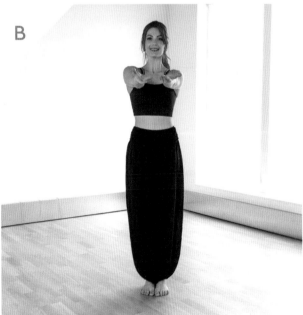

CRISS CROSS

- Stand tall, extend your arms out to the sides at shoulder height, palms facing downward. Now bring your arms forward and criss-cross them in front of your body (first right over left, then left over right), before returning them back past the original position so that you feel the stretch in your upper back muscles. (A) (B)
- Bring your arms forward again, repeating this as many times as you can in 60 seconds before lowering both arms to your sides.

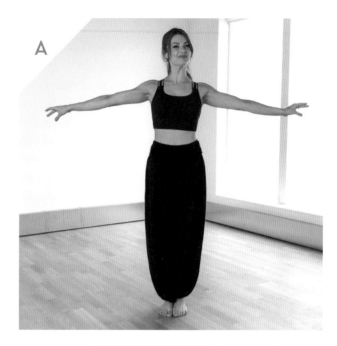

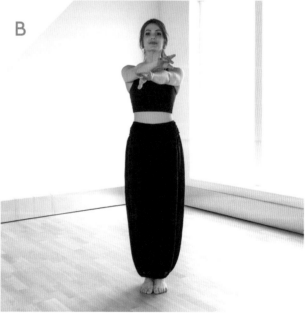

UP AND DOWN

- Stand tall and slowly raise your arms forward to shoulder height and then on up toward the ceiling, keeping your elbows soft and palms turned inward – so that your arms form a slightly rounded shape. **(A) (B)**
- Hold them there briefly before lowering them back down to your sides.
- Repeat as many time as you can in 60 seconds.

A

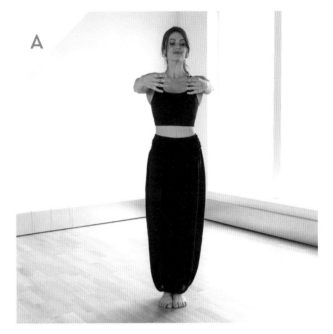

B

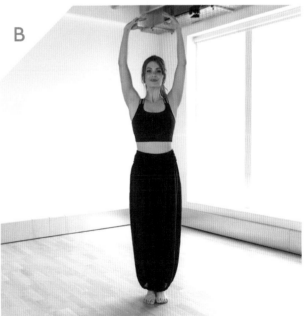

BALLET – CALF RAISES

These simple rise-and-lower moves are a great way to stretch and warm up the muscles in your lower legs; tight calf muscles are always tricky for a dancer.

- Stand tall with your feet slightly apart and rise up onto the balls of both your feet. Hold your arms in a rounded position, with elbows slightly bent. Hold the position for as long as possible and then lower down again slowly and with control. Repeat this as many times as you can in 60 seconds. (A) (B)

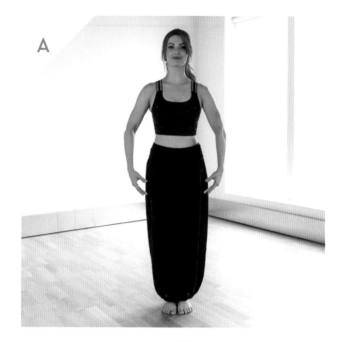

A

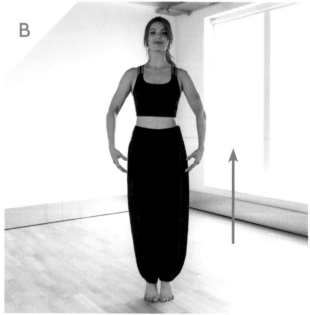

B

- Next, start a single calf raise by raising your right leg so that your right foot is slightly behind your left knee and your right knee is slightly bent in front of you. Then raise up onto the ball of your standing foot before lowering down slowly. **(C) (D)**
- Then do the same thing on the other leg.
- Repeat for 60 seconds on each side.

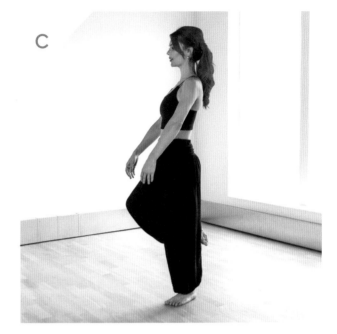

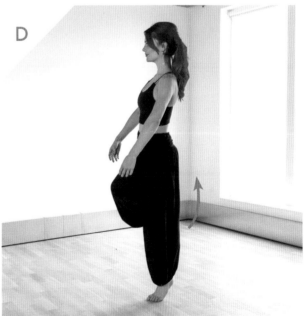

BALLET – PLIÉ SQUAT

Plié means "bent" in French, so a "plié" is a simple knee bend move, which works the thigh and glute muscles to the max. The key is to keep your back upright while doing it, avoiding either leaning backward or forward.

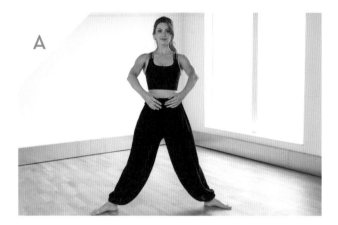

A

- Stand with your feet in a wide stance, pointing your toes outward in a "V" shape, with your arms slightly in front of you in a rounded position at waist height. Your back and legs should be straight, with your stomach muscles engaged and lifted. (A)

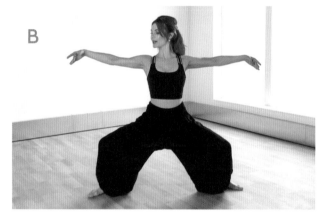

B

- Lower down into a deep squat position, keeping your knees over your feet, raising your arms out to your sides at shoulder height, and either looking straight ahead or letting your head look naturally to one side or the other. Hold for a slow count of five seconds. Don't go down so far that you need to lift your heels off the floor – everyone's plié will look different so just do what suits your body. (B)

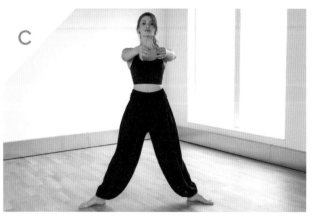

C

- Then push down through your feet to rise up to straight legs again, allowing your arms to move forward as if you are giving someone a hug. (C)
- Repeat the previous two steps as many times as you can in 60 seconds.

TOP TIP

Feel free to hold on to the back of a stable chair – rather than moving the arms – if it helps with balance.

BALLET – PLIÉ SQUAT WITH "SERVING FOOD" ARMS

Let's have a bit of fun now by combining two of the moves that you've already learned – the leg and body action of the Plié Squat with the arms of Serving Food.

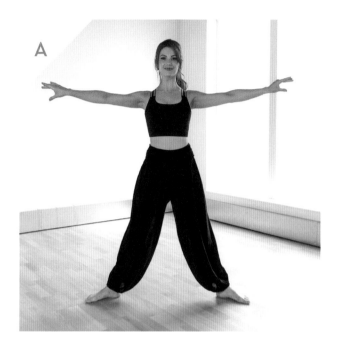

A

- As in the basic Plié Squat exercise (see page 62), stand with your feet in a wide stance, pointing your toes outward in a "V" shape, but, this time, raise your arms out to the sides at shoulder height, palms facing down. (A)
- As you bend your knees outward over your feet to slowly lower yourself into your Plié Squat, with an upright back, move your arms forward and turn your palms upward – so that they are in the final Serving Food position (see page 57). (B)
- Then straighten your legs to come back to upright, raising your arms back out to the sides at shoulder height, palms downward, as you do so.
- Repeat this as many times as you can in 60 seconds, taking two beats to lower and two beats to come up again each time.

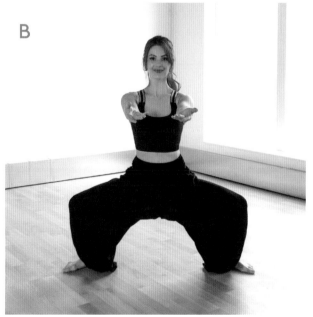

B

TOP TIP

Be sure to let your upper thigh muscles do the work in this controlled dip and rise – *not* your knees.

BALLET – FIRST TO SECOND POSITION SQUAT JUMP

This is more of a cardio move to get your heart pumping as you jump from a narrow squat to a wide one and back again.

- With your feet in First Position – heels together and toes angled outward in a wide "V" shape – bend your knees into a squat stance, keeping your upper body upright. Hold your arms in a rounded position, with elbows slightly bent. Then push yourself upward, jumping off the floor with both feet pointed, and stretch out both legs to land in Second Position – feet still pointing outward but legs in a much wider stance. **(A) (B) (C)**

A
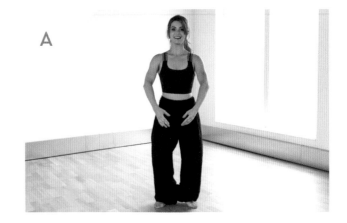

B
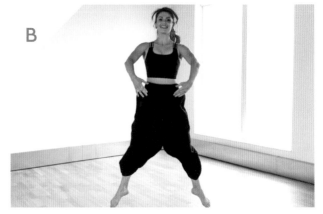

C
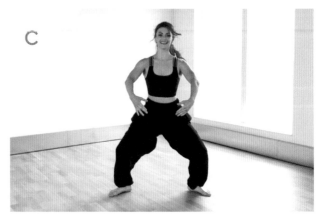

- Then bend your knees into a squat position in this wider stance, launch up into the air and bring both feet back inward to land in First Position again. **(D) (E) (F)**
- Do as many squat jumps as you can in 60 seconds.

TOP TIP

Be sure to land the jumps as lightly as possible by really engaging your leg and bottom muscles (glutes) as you do them.

D
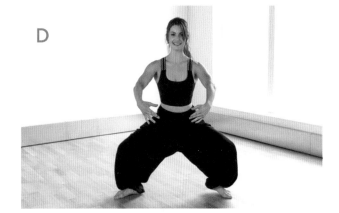

E
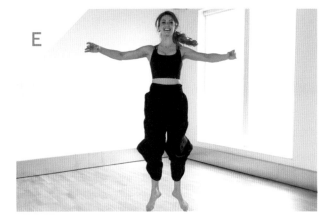

F
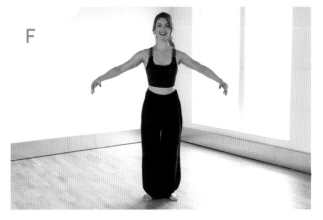

BALLET – CURTSY SQUAT

This is a great move that is neither quite a squat nor a lunge and that will really wake up your inner thighs and glutes!

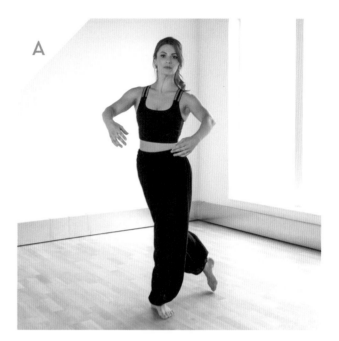

A

- Stand with your feet hip-width apart and your core engaged. Step back with your right leg, placing your right foot behind and to the left of your left foot, and raising your arms out in front of you, keeping your elbows soft to make a nice rounded shape. **(A)**
- Then start to lower yourself into a "curtsy" so that your right knee moves down toward the floor just past your left heel. As you do this, bring your arms up above your head, keeping them rounded rather than straight. If you feel comfortable, continue into a deeper curtsy so that your left leg is bent at a right angle, with your knee almost touching the floor. **(B)**

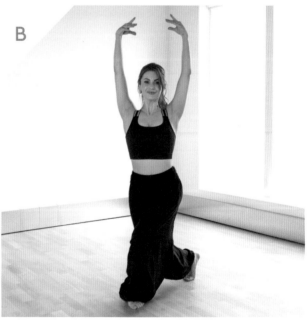

B

- Next, return to standing with your feet hip-width apart, bringing your arms back down to the rounded front position. Then repeat the curtsy on your other leg – this time taking your left leg behind and past your right foot, and lowering your left knee toward the floor by your right foot.
- Repeat for 60 seconds on each side.

TOP TIP
Keep your upper body upright and your shoulders back, rather than hunching over.

BALLET – LYING SPINE TWIST

This is a great back tension reliever and I often use it as a warm-up or cool-down move, as it feels just so great.

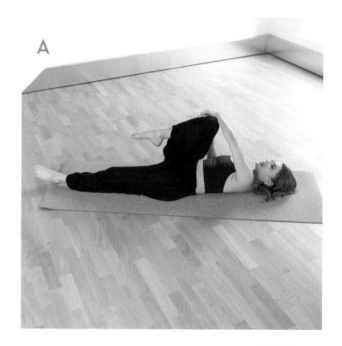

A

- Lie on your back with your legs together on the floor and your arms down by your sides, then hug your right knee up to your chest. (A)
- Using your left hand, gently press your right knee across your body and down toward the floor on your left side, while keeping the left buttock on the floor and the left leg long. Keep your right arm stretched to the side. As you do so, look to the right. Hold the stretch for 30 seconds. (B)
- Return to centre and repeat on the other side.

TOP TIP
Be sure to keep both shoulder blades flat on the mat while you do this.

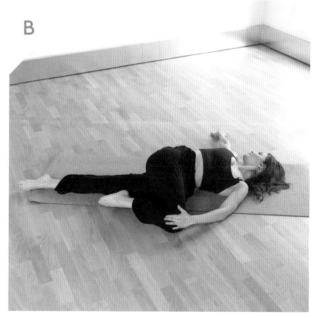

B

BALLET – STANDING LEG LIFTS

Leg lifts really work your core as you control the movement. Each leg lift, alternatively called a *grand battement*, also fires up your thigh muscles and glutes. Feel free to place a chair beside you and hold onto the back of it to help with your balance.

- From standing with your feet together, turn your right foot slightly outward, point it out in front of you and raise your arms out to the sides toward shoulder height, keeping your elbows soft so that you make a nice rounded shape with your arms. **(A)**
- Then lift your right leg directly up in front of you as high as is comfortable while keeping your spine straight, before bringing your foot back to the starting position and tapping the floor lightly with it. **(B)**

A

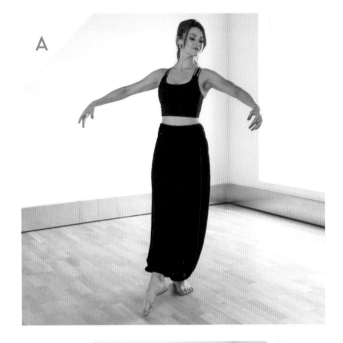

B

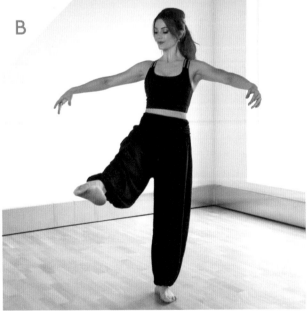

- Next, lift your right leg directly out to the side to a comfortable height, before bringing your foot back to the starting position and tapping the floor lightly with it. **(C)**
- Finally, lift your right leg directly behind you as high as is comfortable, before bringing your foot back to the starting position and tapping the floor lightly with it. **(D)**
- Repeat the lifts – front, side and back – as many times as you can in 60 seconds.
- Then repeat it all on the other side, this time pointing your left leg out in front of you to begin.

TOP TIP

Be sure to keep your standing leg firm as you do the lifts. Your hips should stay parallel for the front and back lifts, and open for the side lift.

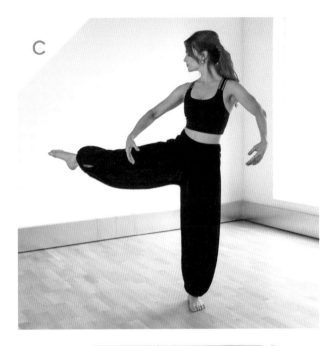

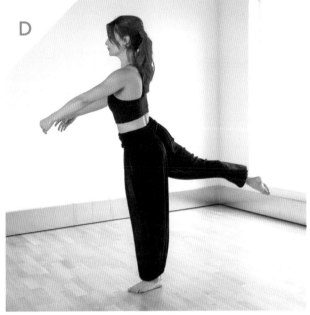

SALSA - BASIC STEP

To get going with the fiery salsa, here's the basic move, which should be done with a lot of energy and a *lot* of hip action! Count the beats in your head to help you keep the rhythm.

- Start with your feet close together and your weight on your left leg. **(A)**
- Step backward with your right foot (beat 1), shifting your weight to this leg. **(B)** Then, transfer your weight onto your front leg (beat 2). **(C)**

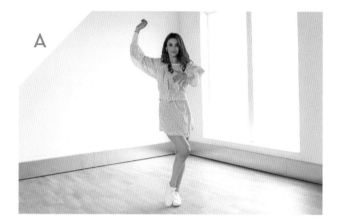

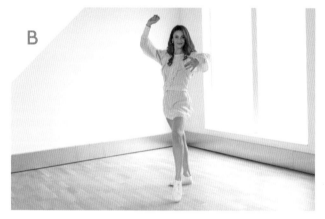

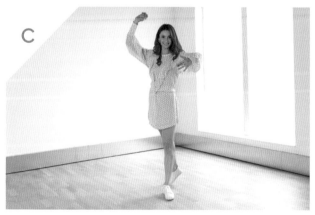

- Next, bring your right foot back to the starting position beside your left foot (beat 3). **(D)**

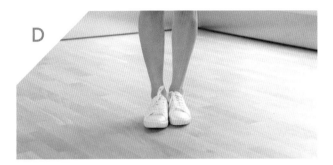

- Hold your position (beat 4). Step forward with your left foot (beat 5), shifting your weight onto your left leg. **(E)** Then, transfer your weight onto your back leg (beat 6) and bring your left foot to the starting position (beat 7). **(F) (G)** Hold the beat (beat 8).

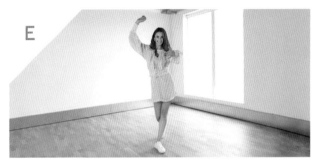

- Repeat as many times as you like, trying the move at both faster and slower tempos. Remember to make sure the tempos are quick, quick, slow ... quick, quick, slow ...

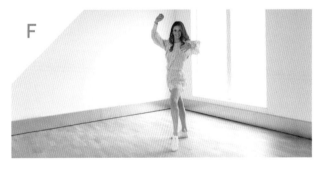

TOP TIP

Salsa was born in packed, steamy Cuban and Puerto Rican dance clubs, so there's no need to move far with these steps – you can keep them nice and small. Once you have the basic technique mastered, you can start to incorporate your head, shoulders and arms, really swinging into the movement as you transfer your weight onto each leg.

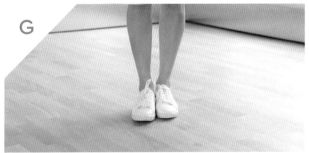

SALSA – BASIC SIDE-STEP

Once you've got the hang of the Basic Step, this side-step should come easily as it's the same move but from side to side, rather than back and forward. Again, count the beats in your head to help you keep the rhythm.

- Start with your feet close together and your weight on your left leg. **(A)** Step your right foot out to the side (beat 1), shifting your weight to this leg. **(B)**
- Transfer your weight to your left leg (beat 2). **(C)**. Bring your right foot back to its starting position (beat 3). **(D)**

A
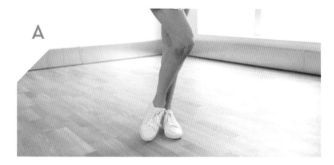

B
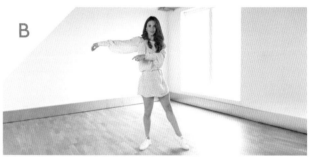

C
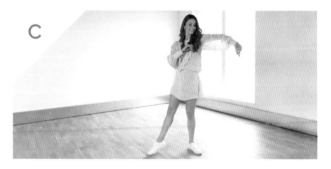

D
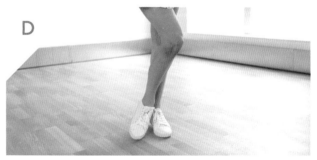

- Now, step your left foot out to the side (beat 4), shifting your weight to this leg. Then, transfer your weight back to your right leg (beat 5). **(E) (F)** Bring your left foot back to its starting position (beat 6). **(G)**
- Repeat as many times as you like, trying the move at both faster and slower tempos. Work in some arm movements when you are ready! Just like the Basic Step, the tempo should be quick, quick, slow ...

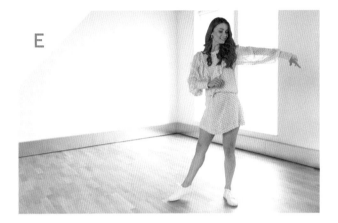

E

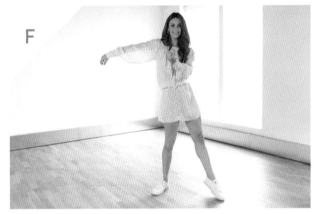

F

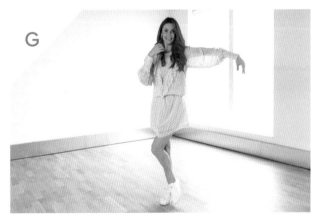

G

SALSA – ZULU

I love this Brazilian dance step that really lets you swing those hips as you march on the spot but with your feet nice and wide, and your arms swinging.

- Start with your feet wider than shoulder-width apart. Step your left foot out to the side, transferring your weight onto your left leg. At the same time, swing your right arm forward and your left arm back. **(A) (B)**
- Then switch, stepping your right foot out to the side and transferring your weight onto your right leg. This time swing your left arm forward and your right arm back. **(C) (D)**
- Repeat the movement, lifting the left foot again and swinging the left arm forward.

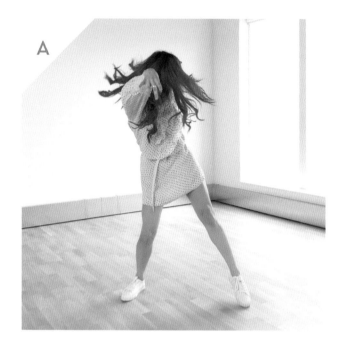

A

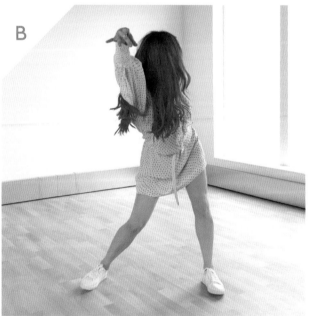

B

- Repeat the same pattern but this time starting on your right foot, with your right arm swinging forward.
- Once you feel comfortable with the movements, you can use the weight of your full body to add extra swing to each "lift", turning your head in a relaxed way to whichever side you're stepping.
- Continue with this alternating Zulu move, doing it as many times as you like.

TOP TIP

As with all these dance moves, hearing the rhythm in your head is so helpful. So put some salsa music on and get moving – the steps don't have to be perfect!

C

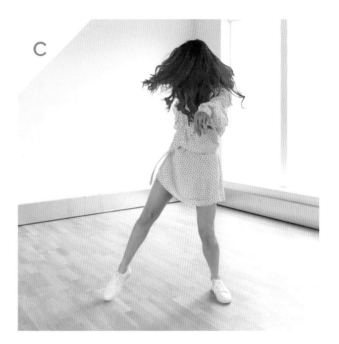

D

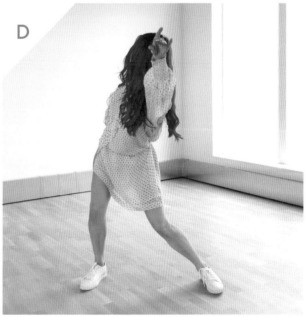

SALSA – SPOT TURN

Why not throw in a Spot Turn as part of your Salsa moves? This is a simple swivel turn that will add an extra sense of dynamism to your dancing. Again, it's useful to count the beats in your head as you do it to help you get into the swing of it.

- Start with your feet close together and your weight on your left leg. (A) Step backward with your right foot (beat 1), shifting your weight back to your right leg and letting your arms move naturally as you get into the salsa vibe! (B)
- Transfer your weight to your front leg (beat 2). (C)
- Bring your right foot back to the starting position beside your left foot (beat 3). (D)

A
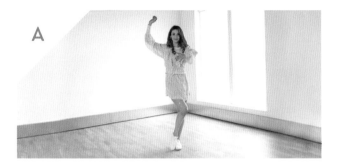

B
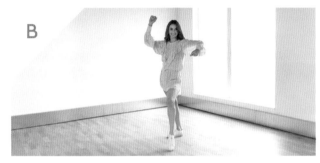

C
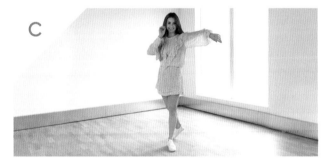

D
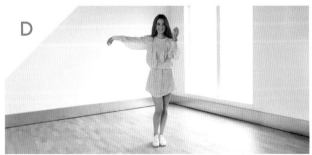

- Step forward with your left foot and shift your weight to this leg (beat 4). **(E)** At this point, imagine that you've hit a wall and can't go any further, so you swivel your feet 180 degrees, shifting your weight to your right foot (beat 5). **(F)**
- Now, step forward and shift your weight forward on your right foot (beat 6). **(G)** Then make half a turn (180 degrees) back to the starting position. **(H)** Close your feet together (beat 7) and hold (beat 8).
- Repeat the move as many times as you like!

TOP TIP

The trick here is to balance your weight on the ball of the turning foot and push off on your spin with the other foot. It might take a little practice! Try to keep your body upright and eyes straight ahead as you do the turns, too.

E
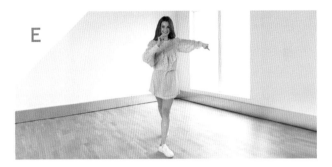

F
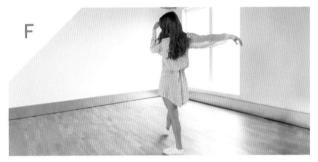

G
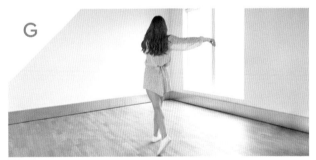

H
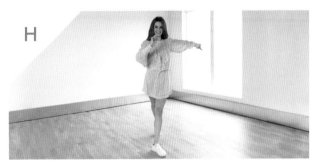

JIVE – FORWARD AND SIDE KICKS

If you've watched jive before, you'll know why I've selected it for the book. It's great fun – energetic and full of clever footwork. We start with a kick step – a simple flicky kick out to the front and then the side. When doing this, always keep a slight bend in your standing leg and both knees soft.

- Stand with your feet slightly less than hip-width apart and hop onto your left leg so that your right foot is lifted off the floor and your right knee is bent. **(A)**
- Then, kick your right foot forward in a swift movement, pointing your toes, before drawing your right leg back up to its bent starting position. That's a forward kick! **(B)**

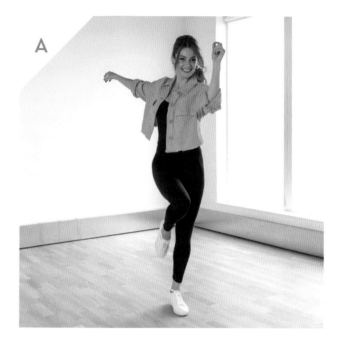

A

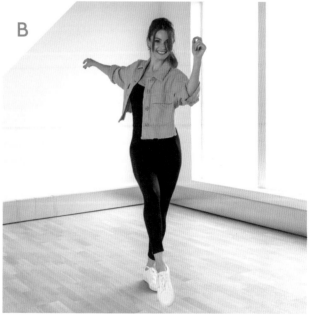

B

- For a side kick, from the same starting position (C), simply kick your right foot out to the side, pointing your toes as you do so (D), and pull it back again quickly.
- Combine these moves by flowing straight from the right front kick (Step 1) to the right side kick (Step 2).
- Then hop onto your right leg and do the same two kicks with your left leg.

TOP TIP

The jive involves lots of kicks and flicks, so to keep your balance, shift your weight on to the balls of your feet, bend your knees a little and lean your upper body forward slightly, with your pelvis tipped backward. Once you've got the hang of it, you can move your arms along with the movement in whatever way feels most natural for you.

C

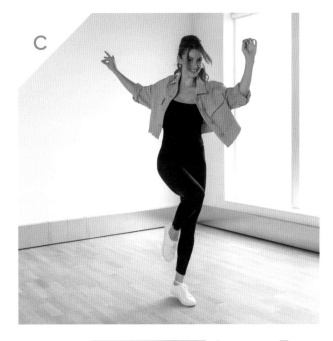

D

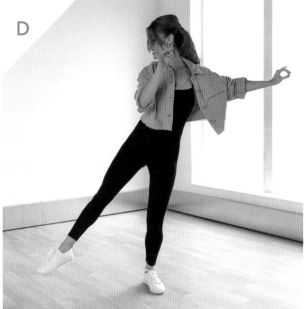

JIVE – CHASSÉ

One of the most common jive moves, the Chassé is a satisfying "chasing" side-step that moves you across the floor. Think side-step, together, side-step, together and relax into it with a little bounce and some hip action.

- Starting with your feet slightly less than hip-width apart, step out with your right foot and then "hop" your left foot over and down to meet it. Then repeat the movement, again starting with your right foot. (A) (B)

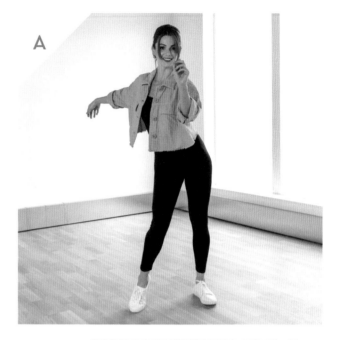

A

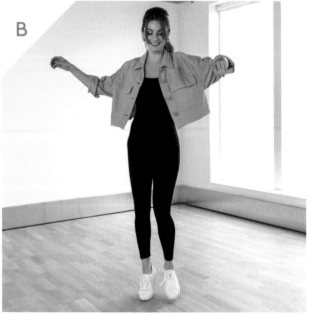

B

- Then, step out with your left foot and "hop" your right foot to meet it. Repeat this movement again on the left side. **(C)**
- As you continue the chassé, move from side to side, gradually speeding it up, keeping on the balls of your feet to bring some height into the step. **(D)**
- Once you've figured out the footwork, add your arms in opposition to your feet, stretching your left arm forward as you move your right foot to the side.
- Repeat the move on alternate sides for as long as you would like.

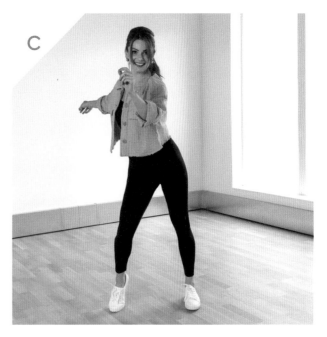

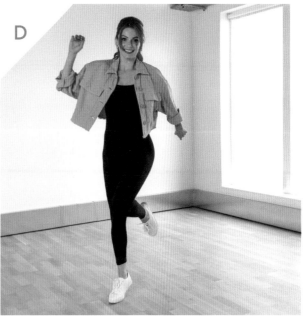

JIVE – TOE HEEL STEP

Now you've mastered a couple of key basic jive moves, here's a more dynamic step with some swinging action as you cross your legs. Take this at whatever speed feels most comfortable for you.

- Starting with your feet slightly less than hip-width apart, lift your right foot and tap your toes against the floor just in front of your left leg, with your foot angled slightly inward. **(A)**
- Then, rotate your foot so that it is angled outward and tap your heel against the floor. **(B)**

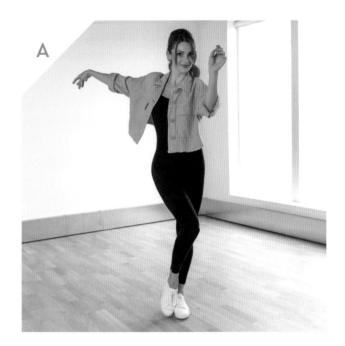

A

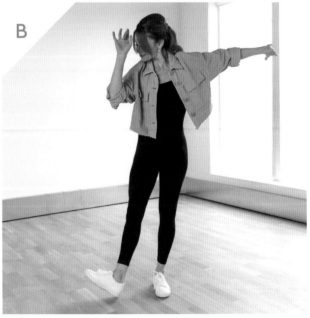

B

- Step your right foot to the left of your left foot, transferring your body weight onto your right foot as you do so, and lifting your left leg off the floor in readiness to do the whole move on the other side. **(C)**
- This time, tap the toes of your left foot, angled slightly inward, against the floor just in front of your right leg. Then, tap your left heel to the floor so that it is angled outward, finally stepping your left foot on the floor to the right of your right foot. **(D)**
- Repeat the move on alternate sides, letting your arms swing naturally with the movement for as long as you like.

TOP TIP

This is a "swing" style of dancing so aim to let your rib cage and hips lead the movement.

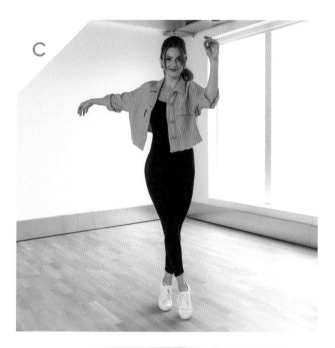

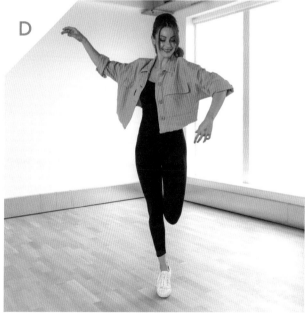

JIVE – JUMP BACK WITH CLAP

Our final jive move is a simple jump backward followed by a clap. This should be a short shunt backward – don't try to jump too far. It's almost like a little twerk as you jump back – so "twerk, clap, twerk, clap"!

- Stand with your feet wider than hip-width apart and your knees slightly bent. **(A)**
- Jump back a small distance, raising and extending your arms outward at shoulder height as you do so. **(B)**
- Once you've landed, give an emphatic clap to finish the movement, or as a break before the next jump back if you're doing several in succession. **(C)**
- Repeat this Jump Back with Clap as many times as it takes you to feel comfortable with it.

TOP TIP

Don't jump too far or too high, so that you can keep the tempo up once you're doing it in time to music.

A
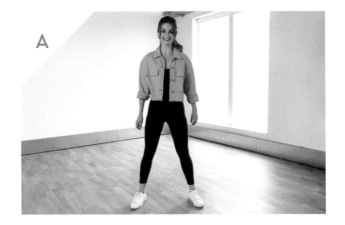

B
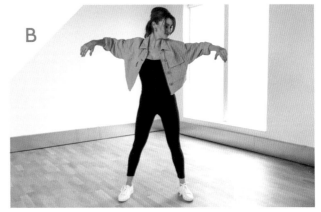

C
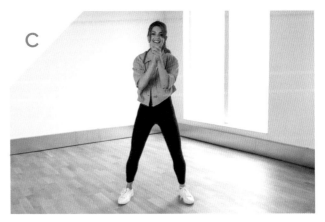

TAP – BALL HEEL

We start the tap section with a simple "ball heel" move. In tap, you use either the ball or the heel of your foot to tap the floor – and when one is done after the other, it creates a two-sound "tap, tap" move.

- Start with your feet slightly less than hip-width apart. Shift your weight onto your left leg and lift your right foot very slightly off the floor. **(A)** Quickly "tap" the floor with the ball of your right foot, keeping your heel up. **(B)** Then tap the floor with the heel of your right foot as you lower the rest of your foot. **(C)**
- To repeat the step on your other foot, shift your weight onto your right leg as you raise your left foot off the floor. Tap the ball of your left foot down, keeping the heel up. Finally tap the heel of your left foot down as you lower the rest of your foot.
- Continue the move by alternating it on each foot.

TOP TIP

Always keep your knees "soft" in tap (i.e. slightly bent) to make it easier to transfer your weight between your feet as you tap one foot at a time.

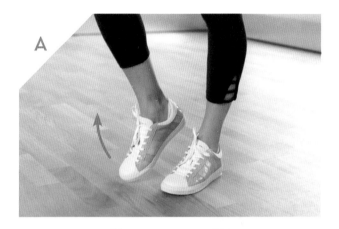

A

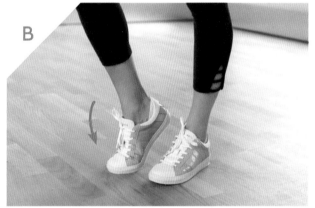

B

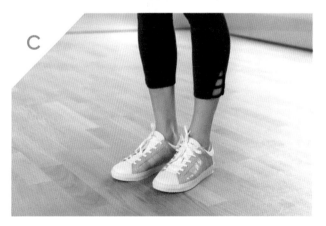

C

TAP – SHUFFLE TAP

The shuffle is another key tap move – also known as the "brush". In this one, you "brush" or "scuff" the floor with the ball of your foot without putting the rest of your foot down. It's a bit like the previous tap move, but you bring your foot up again as soon as you've made the sound, instead of placing the rest of your foot down. The full move should make a three-part "scuff, scuff, tap" sound.

- Stand with your feet slightly less than hip-width apart.
- Placing your weight over your left foot and side, bend your right knee and lift your right foot a short way off the floor. (A) Quickly brush the ball of your right foot against the floor as you swing your leg forward from the knee. Note that the heel of the right foot doesn't touch the floor as you do this. (B) (C)

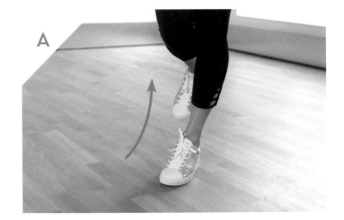

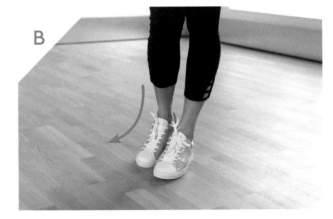

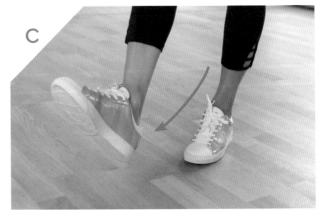

- Then brush the ball of the same foot a second time against the floor, this time as you swing your leg backwards, bending the lower leg slightly up behind as you do so. (D) (E) Finally, lower your foot to the floor beside the other one in a single stop movement, creating a "tap". (F)
- To repeat on the other side, transfer your weight onto your right leg and brush the ball of your left foot forward and then backward against the floor in a swinging action. Practise doing this until it feels natural and you can do it quickly while holding your balance on the standing leg.

TOP TIP

As tap dancing involves switching balance between your feet quickly and often, it's helpful to keep your weight mainly over the balls of your feet.

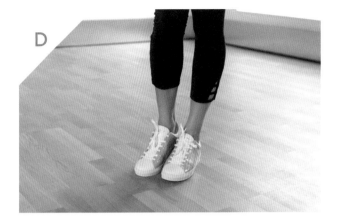

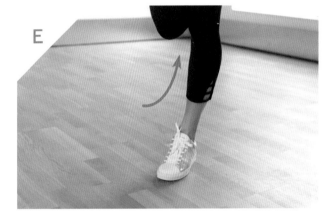

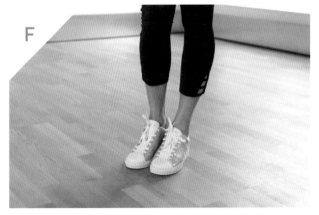

TAP – SHUFFLE BALL HEEL

Now we're going to do the shuffle ball heel, one leg at a time. A shuffle step is a brush of one foot forward, followed by the two-part placement of the same foot back down on the floor – firstly the ball, then the heel ("tap, tap"). Hence there being three sounds to one shuffle step: "scuff, tap, tap".

- Stand with your feet slightly less than hip-width apart. **(A)**
- Placing your weight over your left foot, lift your right foot slightly off the floor. **(B)** Swing your right foot forward, brushing the ball against the floor to make a "scuff" sound. **(C) (D)**

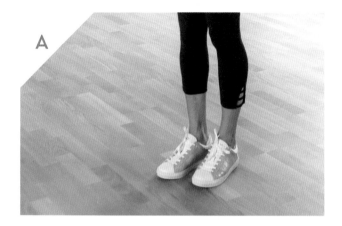

A

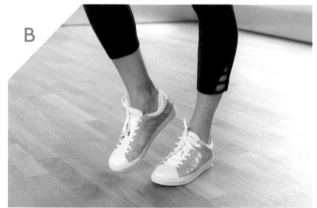

B

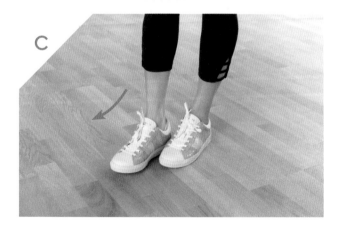

C

- Place down the ball of your right foot onto the floor in front of you, then the heel, so that your foot ends up flat on the floor in front of you. **(E) (F)** This ball–heel placement creates the "tap, tap".
- To do the move on the other foot, shift your weight to your right foot and swing your left foot forward – brushing the ball against the floor to make a "scuff" sound. Then lower it to the floor in front of you using the same ball-heel movement as in the previous step ("tap, tap").
- Do this "shuffle step" move on alternate sides, practising until it feels natural to move this way and you can do it at speed.

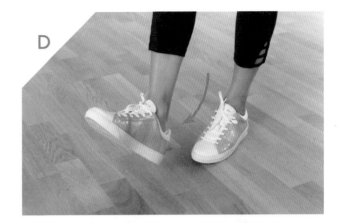

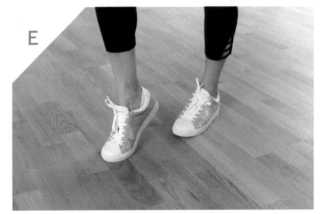

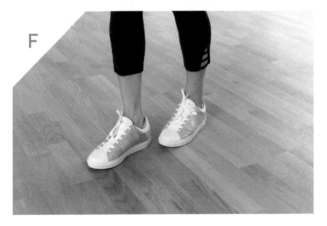

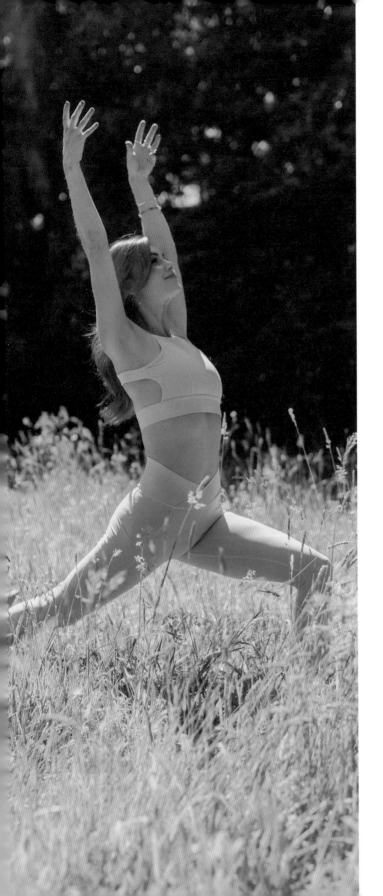

PILATES EXERCISES TO STRENGTHEN AND SCULPT

To me, Pilates is a more "scientific" approach to movement than dance, which might make it sound tricky, but it's actually a wonderful way to understand more about how your body works and learn simple movements and stretches that will make it stronger, more flexible and improve how it functions.

Pilates was first introduced to me by my ballroom and Latin dance coach when I was in my late twenties. She would make us do Pilates at every single session before we started dancing and I was soon hooked. I feel more "dance-y" when I'm doing my yoga, but with Pilates, I feel that I'm working on *all* parts of my body.

Pilates was recommended to me specifically to improve my core strength and posture. I was in a show and my teacher said it would teach me how to properly engage my core and straighten my spine. At the time, I wasn't focused on its all-round health benefits; I saw it as a tool to simply improve my dancing.

Boxers and Ballerinas

Unlike yoga with its long history in Eastern philosophy, Pilates is a relatively modern form of exercise. Joseph "Joe" Pilates was born in 1880 in Germany and, after a childhood blighted by poor health, he studied anatomy and became a gymnast and boxer with an interest in yoga and bodybuilding. At the beginning of World War I, he was living as a boxer in England and was interned due to his nationality. In the camp, he devised an exercise regime to help rehabilitate injured soldiers returning from battle. When he returned to Germany after the war, he was then asked to help the German army with strength training but chose to move to the US, where he set up a studio in New York training boxers. Rumour has it that there were some dance studios in the same building and that the ballerinas began to visit him to learn techniques to help them strengthen their bodies, and to both ease and avoid aches and strains.

His Pilates method is a system of movements and stretches designed to improve strength, mobility and flexibility, as well as to build a strong core, which influences so many other aspects of the body.

When I started doing it, I quickly found that the simple, controlled moves had a powerful effect on my body, strengthening and lengthening my muscles and making me walk taller. My teacher would pull my shoulders back and tell me that "If we get your back a little stronger, your glutes will work better, and so on." Because it's all connected – the power of strong glutes works its way up the body, making the back stronger and the lats (*latissimus dorsi* – major back muscles on each side of the body) move down, improving overall posture.

A dance teacher of mine used to tell me to imagine that I had a kebab stick up the middle of the body, from my feet all the way to my head, when I was dancing. The stick should always stay straight but the body can rotate all its parts around it. Pilates helps me to understand and remember this idea of keeping the body "stacked" and aligned, with the posture straight and tall.

Core Strength

Your core is at the heart of Pilates work – a strong middle section (or "powerhouse" in the Pilates world) influences the rest of the body. As a dancer, I'm thinking of lots of aspects of movement at the same time so don't focus on the core as strongly, but, in Pilates, the movement is slow, controlled and focused. More than just ab exercises, Pilates works on the deep middle muscles that affect the back, hip and abdominal muscles – the ones that impact posture, balance your body (we tend to favour one side of our body over the other) and enable easy movement, including bending and lifting. Basically, Pilates is key to optimal everyday movement, whether it's correcting your desk-slouching habit or building strength for carrying heavy bags of shopping.

Many of us don't know how to properly engage our core muscles. I was taught to engage mine by lying on my back with my knees bent and my feet on the floor, just breathing. As you breathe in, you let your stomach fully expand and your rib cage move outward. Then as you breathe out, you let your stomach contract and draw your belly button toward your rib cage, feeling your core muscles in your abdomen and your sides contract. Without holding your breath, you then keep the core muscles in that position.

I still do this exercise with my students. Just getting someone to lie down and engage their core, then do a simple sit-up – a very basic move – tells you a lot. Many people use their *neck* for the sit-up, instead of their *core*. So try using your *core* to do a slow sit-up – and repeating this five times. Then, from your position lying on your back with your knees bent and feet on the floor, try lifting up both your legs, keeping them straight, before bringing them back down, tapping the floor with your heels and raising them again five times. It sounds quite simple but, done properly, it will make you sweat.

Equipment and Benefits

Pilates can be done by anyone, with or without gym experience, and with just a mat, but you'll find that many classes also use a few key Pilates tools. Pilates rings are, for example, good for strength exercises. These are circular rings that you can use to add pressure to moves for your arms and legs; I use them when I want to add a little more oomph to a move. And resistance bands are stretchy lengths of elastic fabric that are useful to add tension to certain moves if you're a little more experienced.

Joseph Pilates once said: "After 10 hours of Pilates, you'll feel a difference. After 20 hours, you'll see a difference. After 30 hours, you'll have a new body."

"After 10 hours of Pilates, you'll feel a difference. After 20 hours, you'll see a difference. After 30 hours, you'll have a new body."

Joseph Pilates

PILATES EXERCISES

1. Neutral Position and Pelvic Tilt
2. Side Lunge
3. Ragdoll with Swing
4. High Lunge with Cactus Arms
5. Side Plank
6. Half Splits
7. Plank
8. Oblique Curl
9. Tabletop Arms and Legs
10. Dead Bug
11. Lying Leg Circles
12. Corkscrew
13. Lying Leg Scissor Kicks
14. Double Straight Leg Stretch
15. Bridge Pose
16. Reverse Bridge with Leg Lift
17. Donkey Kicks
18. Mountain Climbers
19. Hip Rolls
20. Knees to Chest

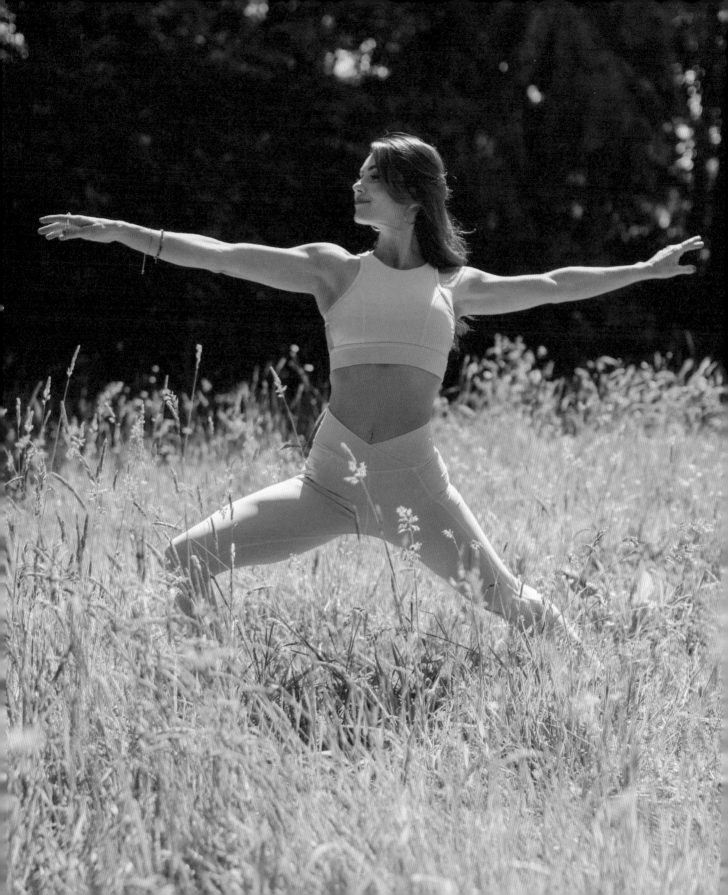

NEUTRAL POSITION AND PELVIC TILT

Before we start looking at the Pilates moves properly, I want to show you the common positions of the pelvis in Pilates – an awareness of which will make all the difference when it comes to doing the poses themselves.

- **Neutral position:** Lie on the mat with your knees bent, feet flat on the floor and arms by your sides. Be aware of your shoulders, rib cage and tailbone against the mat, and keep your spine long. In this neutral position, your lower back will have a very slight natural curve. **(A)**
- **Pelvic tilt:** Again, lying on the mat with your knees bent and your feet flat on the floor, press your lower spine flat against the floor, lifting your tailbone lightly and tilting your pelvis toward you. **(B)** Then reverse this move by tilting your pelvis away from you and bringing an arch to the lower back. **(C)** If it helps, think of a ball placed on your belly button – with the *first* tilt you are trying to roll the ball toward your head, with the *second* you are trying to roll it toward your feet.

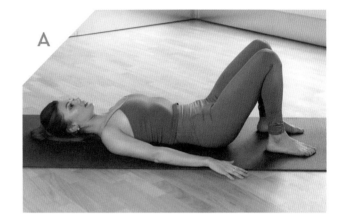

A

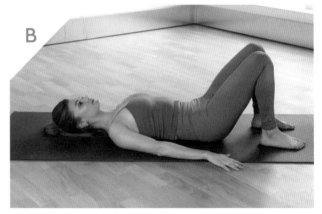

B

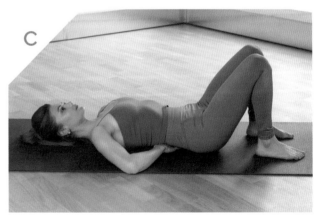

C

SIDE LUNGE

Also known as a lateral lunge, this is a great move for your leg muscles and glutes. It is a particularly useful tool to help strengthen the body for sideways movements, too.

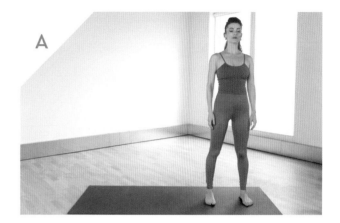

- Stand sideways on the mat with your feet hip-width apart and engage your core, then step out with your right foot to a wide stance, with your feet pointing diagonally outward. **(A) (B)**
- On an inhale, bend your right knee into a right-angle lunge, keeping your left leg straight and both feet flat on the floor, with the toes of your left foot facing forward while the toes of your right foot face diagonally outward. If you feel comfortable, bring your hands together into prayer position at your chest. **(C)**
- On an exhale, use your right leg to push you back upright to the original position. Do this 5 times.
- Repeat the exercise on the other side.

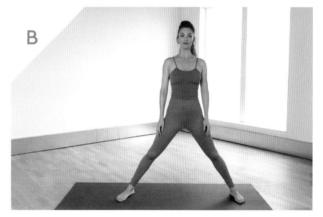

TOP TIP
Focus on the thigh muscles doing the work during this movement, rather than the knees.

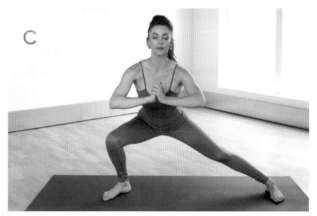

RAGDOLL WITH SWING

Often a warm-up or cool-down pose, this lovely freeing forward bend really opens up the lower back and stretches your hamstrings and calf muscles.

- Stand tall on the mat with your feet slightly wider than hip-width apart. **(A)**
- Take a deep breath in and, on your next exhale, slowly fold from your waist, letting your arms hang heavy in front of you, until your belly rests against your thighs, or as close as it will reach, keeping your knees slightly bent if this feels more comfortable. **(B)**

A

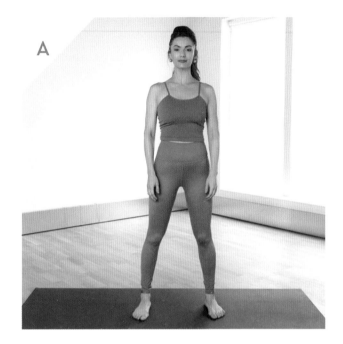

B

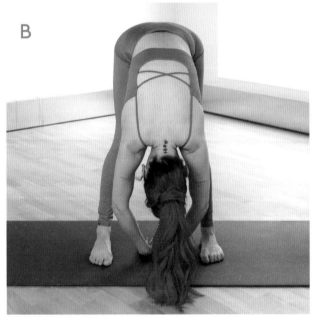

- If comfortable, clasp your opposite elbows with your hands and let your body hang down and enjoy the stretch here for 30 seconds. **(C)**
- Swing gently from side to side to bring some extra movement to the stretch, making sure you're not holding any tension in your head or neck. **(D) (E)**
- Gently roll back up to standing, slowly stacking your spine one vertebra at a time and bringing your head up last.

TOP TIP

Keep your feet firmly rooted to the floor in this move, with your weight as evenly distributed as possible.

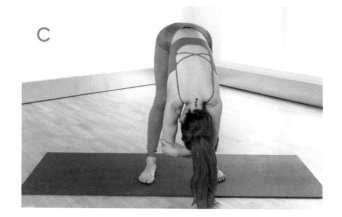

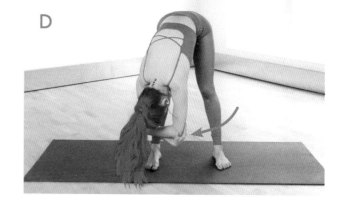

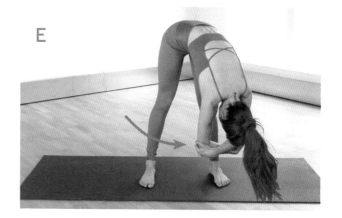

HIGH LUNGE WITH CACTUS ARMS

This lunge pose is a brilliant move for strength, balance and co-ordination, and adding raise "cactus" arms to it opens up your chest area, relieving tension in your upper body. The key is to keep your upper body straight, and focus your energy on your core and the front foot.

- Stand at the front of the mat with your feet together and engage your core. **(A)**
- On an inhale, take a large step backward with your right leg, balancing it on the toes of your right foot. At the same time, bend your left knee into a right angle, keeping that foot flat on the floor, to form a lunge position. Then raise your hands, palms together, to the ceiling. **(B)**

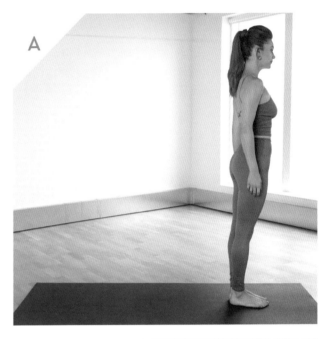

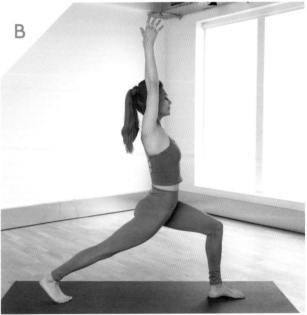

- On an exhale, lower your arms on each side so that they're level with your shoulders, with forearms bent up at right angles and palms facing forward, with fingers spread. Hold the pose for 30 seconds at first, working up to 60 seconds when you feel ready. **(C)**
- Then switch your legs to repeat the move on the other side.

TWIST VARIATION

Add a twist to this pose by turning your upper body in the direction of your forward leg – so twist to the right when your right leg is forward and to the left when your left leg is forward.

LOW LUNGE VARIATION

For a deeper leg stretch, place your back knee on the floor for a low version of this lunge.

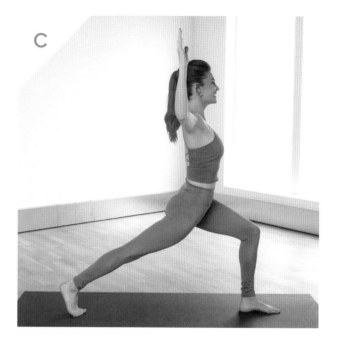

C

SIDE PLANK

This pose targets the side abdominal muscles known as the obliques. The full Side Plank involves supporting your own body weight with a straight arm but it's best to start with this modified version, where you support yourself with a bent arm.

- Start by lying on your right side on the mat, with your body in a straight line, your right arm extended above your head on the floor and your left hand on the floor in front of you for balance. (A)
- Bend your right arm, place the palm of your right hand on the floor slightly in front of your shoulder, fingertips facing forward, and carefully lift your upper body weight onto this arm, ensuring that your elbow is directly under your shoulder. Your left arm can rest along your left side. (B)
- Engage your abdominal muscles and, on your next exhale, raise your hips from the mat so that your body forms a straight line, supported by your elbow. Attempt to hold the position for 30 seconds at first, working up to 60 seconds when you feel ready. (C)
- Rest, then turn over to repeat on your left side.

LIFTING LEG VARIATION

Once steady in the raised position, try lifting your top leg away from your bottom leg for the hold.

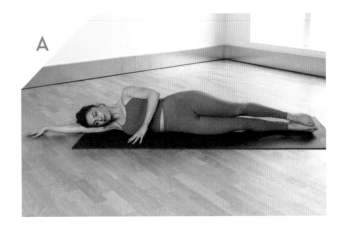

A

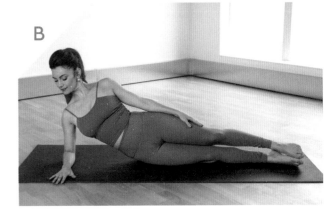

B

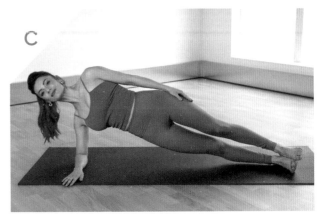

C

HALF SPLITS

A brilliant hip opener and stretch for the hamstrings, this move is particularly useful for dancers and is great preparation for anyone wanting to work on doing the full splits.

- Begin in an upright kneeling position with knees hip-width apart. **(A)**
- Bring your right leg forward in front of you, bending it at a right angle, with your foot flat on the floor. **(B)**
- On an exhale, shift your weight backward onto your left leg, placing your hands on the mat for balance. At the same time, straighten your right leg without locking the knee, and flex your right toes toward your body for 30 seconds. **(C)**
- Then return to an upright kneeling position and switch legs to repeat on the other side.

TOP TIP

Be careful to keep your hips square and not to lean sideways as you do this move.

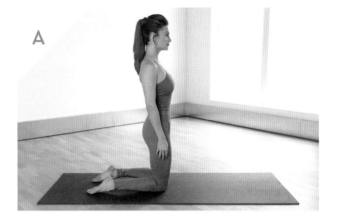

A

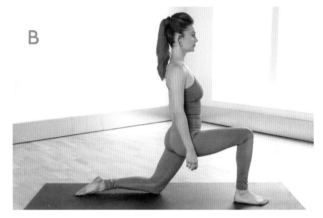

B

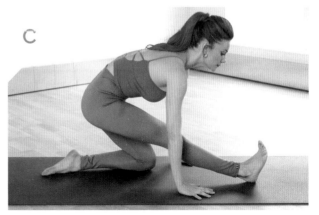

C

PLANK

This foundational pose can help us improve so many of the common movements in Pilates. If you find it difficult, try it on bent knees or elbows – the priority is having a straight line in the body. Then just slowly build up the time you spend in it. The steps below show a Forearm Plank, but if you feel comfortable you can increase the difficulty and do a Straight Arm Plank.

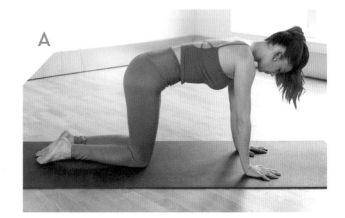

- Begin on all fours on the mat, with your knees hip-width apart and your shoulders over your wrists. Remember to engage your core. **(A)**
- Take your right leg to the back of the mat, using your right toes to balance. **(B)**
- Step your left leg back to join the right, using the strength of your shoulders, arms and core to support your weight. Your body should now make a straight line. Then gently lower yourself one arm at a time onto your forearms if you feel comfortable to do so, with your palms down and fingertips spread wide. Look at the floor slightly ahead of you and breathe naturally. Hold this pose for as long as possible – 30 seconds to start with, if you can. **(C)**

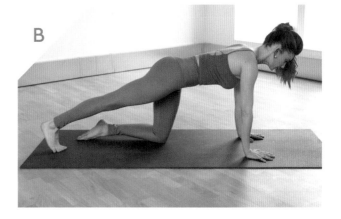

STRAIGHT ARM PLANK VARIATION:
If the forearm position of the supporting arms doesn't feel challenging, try keeping your supporting arms straight (although not locked).

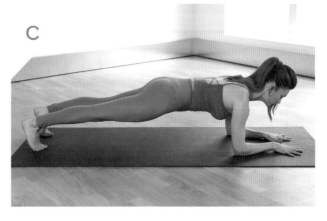

OBLIQUE CURL

This is such a useful move and one that's crucial to do in a controlled manner. You might find it helpful to imagine a glass of water sitting in the centre of your hips as you do it; then try to do the move without spilling a drop!

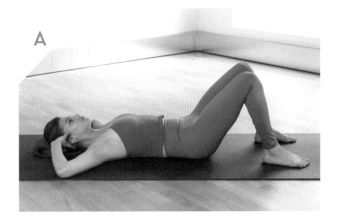

- Lie on your back on the mat with your knees bent and your feet flat on the floor. Place your hands behind your head, elbows wide. Engage your abdominals and ensure that your spine is in a neutral position. **(A)**

- Now, using your core, exhale as you lift your head and neck off the mat. Be sure to use your hands to help support the weight of your head to take pressure off your neck. **(B)**

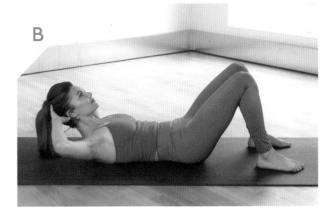

- Next, inhale and twist to the right, keeping your upper body off the floor without closing your elbows in or forcing your head or neck. Feel your rib cage fold toward your hips but make sure to keep your pelvis flat on the floor. Hold this twist for a breath and then come back to the centre position. Repeat this 5 times. **(C)**

- Then do the twist 5 times to your left side.

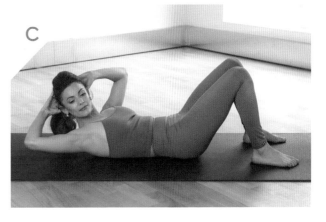

TOP TIP

Keep your elbows wide and out of sight – your oblique muscles should be twisting, not your arms, so that when you lift up you shouldn't be able to see your elbows in your peripheral vision.

TABLETOP ARMS AND LEGS

This pose is a powerhouse move for strengthening the core and pelvic stability. Focus on keeping the core strong and balanced before lifting your limbs slowly and in a controlled manner.

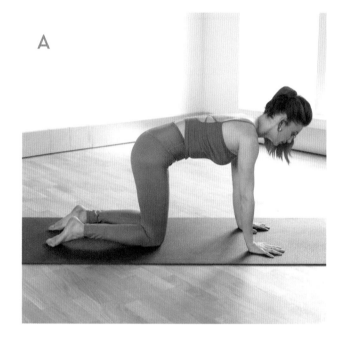

A

- Begin on all fours on the mat, in a "tabletop" position – with your knees bent and hands flat on the floor, both hip-width apart. Ensure that your back is parallel to the floor and long, with your shoulders drawn down away from your ears. Your knees should be under your hips, and your hands beneath your shoulders. **(A)**
- Inhale and lengthen your spine and, as you exhale, lift and extend your right arm and left leg, letting them "float" gently up so that they are straight and in line with the body. Hold this stretch for 10 seconds, keeping the pelvis area stable, then draw your arm and leg back to the starting tabletop position. **(B)**
- Repeat on the other side. Then alternate from one side to the other until you've done 5 on each side.

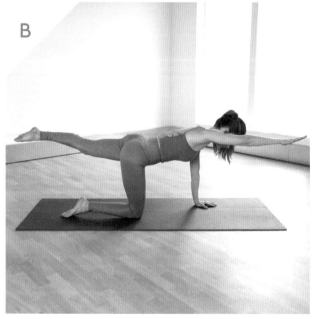

B

TOP TIP
This move is all about alignment – having knees and hips in one line, wrists and shoulders in one line, and a nice flat back before you lift your arms and legs. Use your core to keep the lifts slow and controlled.

DEAD BUG

Many say that this move is better than a plank for the core! It starts from a reverse tabletop position and really works the ab muscles. Start with lifting just your legs if you're a beginner.

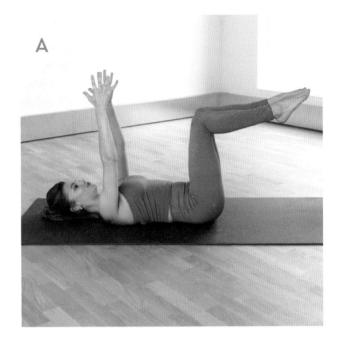

- Lie flat on your back on the mat, with your arms extended up toward the ceiling. Engage your core and draw in your belly button to ensure that your back is not arching. Breathe in while lifting and bending both legs slowly so that your knees are at right angles and your lower legs are parallel with the floor. (A)
- As you exhale, extend and lower your left leg so that it is straight and held just above the floor. At the same time, lower your right arm, extending it backward behind your head so that it is hovering above the floor. (B)
- Inhale and return to the starting position before doing the move on the other side. Then repeat the move 6 times in total, alternating sides.

TOP TIP

Ensure that your core remains engaged, your back is not arching away from the floor and that your shoulders stay on the floor.

KNEE TO ELBOW VARIATION

You can also do this move with your elbows bent and hands behind your head, twisting your shoulder toward your opposite knee.

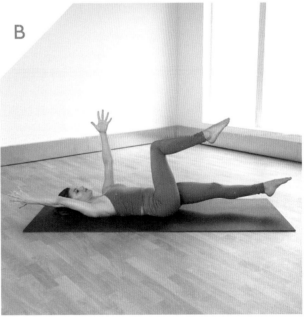

LYING LEG CIRCLES

This is a simple exercise that is more challenging (and good for you) than you may realize! The difficult part is keeping your core still while your hips move. The lower your leg, the more difficult the exercise will be. If you try it with both a pointed foot and a flexed foot, you will work out different parts of your leg. (You might even want to try writing your name with your foot.)

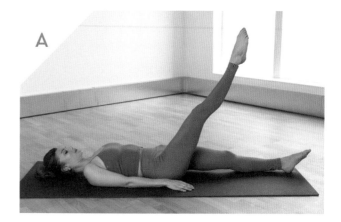

- Lie on your back with straight legs hip-width apart and your arms by your sides, palms facing down. Engage your core and raise your right leg toward the ceiling. **(A)**

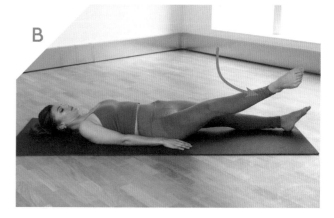

- Breathing naturally, use your toes to slowly draw large and controlled clockwise circles in the air above you. Draw 6 circles in a clockwise direction, then 6 circles in an anti-clockwise direction, ensuring that your lower back stays firmly connected to the floor. **(B) (C)**
- Lower your right leg to the floor and then raise your left leg to draw 6 circles in each direction.

TOP TIP
This should be a controlled movement. If you find your leg is veering out to the side, make your circles smaller.

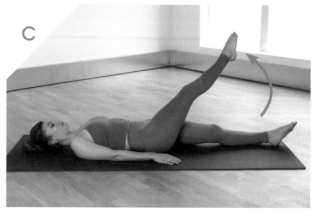

EASIER VARIATION
Bend your leg remaining on the floor so that your foot is flat on the mat.

CORKSCREW

This flowing exercise, which involves moving your legs as if "drawing" a large teardrop shape in the air with your toes, is particularly great for the abdominals, hip and inner thighs.

- Lie on the floor with your legs and feet together and your arms alongside your body, palms down. Now engage your core and raise your legs to the ceiling, keeping your legs straight and pointing your toes. **(A)**

- Then move your legs as if "drawing" a large teardrop shape in the air with your toes – first in a clockwise direction, then in an anti-clockwise direction. Breathe naturally throughout this exercise. The bigger your teardrop is, the more difficult the exercise will be. **(B) (C)**

- Repeat the full teardrop shape 4 times and then another 4 times in the reverse direction before lowering gently back to the floor.

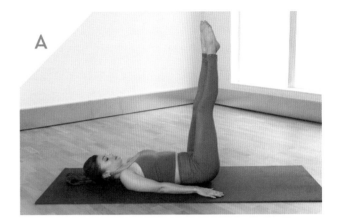

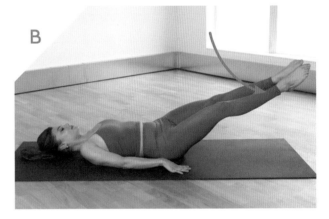

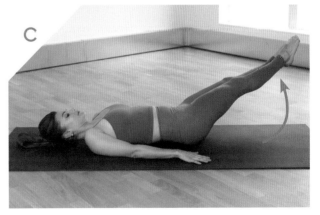

LYING LEG SCISSOR KICKS

There's no denying it – this is a tough move, but I love it! It really works your core and is all about controlled movements while keeping the core and upper body still.

- Start by lying on your back with knees to your chest and your arms wrapped around your legs. Take a deep breath. (A)
- On your exhale, extend both legs up toward the ceiling, moving your arms to lie flat on the floor, palms down, for balance. (B)

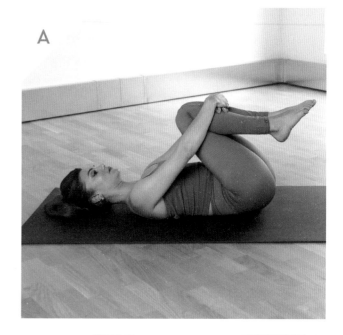

A

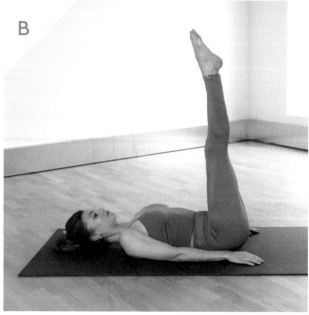

B

- On your inhale, lift your head and neck off the mat – as high as is comfortable – and reach out to lightly hold your right knee, without pulling on it. **(C)**
- On your exhale, lower your left leg until it is hovering just off the mat, keeping it straight. **(D)**
- Pulse the right leg at the top of the lift twice and then switch legs so that your left leg is raised toward you and your right leg is hovering just off the mat. Repeat 5 times on each side.

TOP TIP

Keep your core engaged when you're raising and lowering your legs. And try to extend and lengthen your lower leg in the stretch.

C

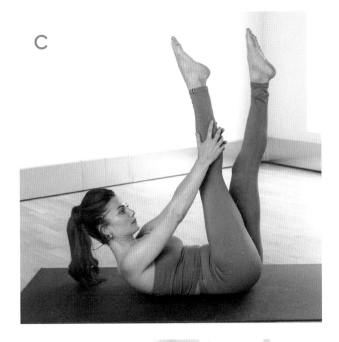

D

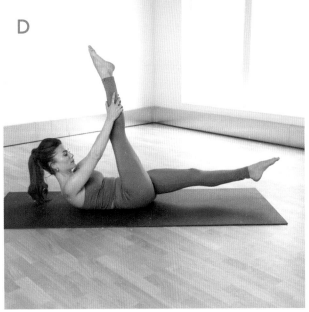

DOUBLE STRAIGHT LEG STRETCH

This is an advanced Pilates move designed to work on your stability and core strength. Work on your technique before your reps for this one, building up your stamina and abdominal co-ordination. You'll feel so satisfied when this move comes together.

- Start by lying on your back with your legs raised and bent at a right angle so that your lower legs are parallel to the mat and your arms are by your side, palms facing down. Engage your abdominal muscles. (A)
- On your inhale, curl your head and shoulders off the mat without straining or pulling your neck. (B)
- Then extend your arms behind you at roughly a 45-degree angle while straightening your legs and holding them at a 45-degree angle to the floor, too. (C)

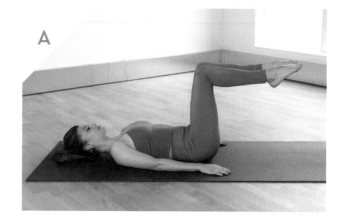

A

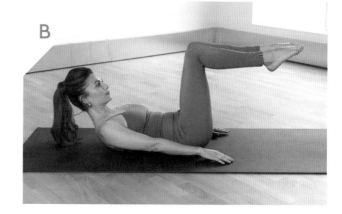

B

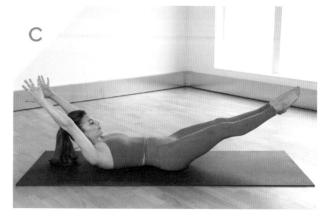

C

- On your exhale, bring your knees toward your face and reach your arms around your legs so that your fingertips touch your ankles, or as near as possible. **(D)**

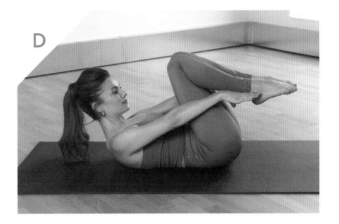

- On your next exhale, stretch your legs away from you again so that they are at a 45-degree angle to the floor and return your arms to their former position, stretching behind you at a 45-degree angle. Repeat this 6 times. **(E)**

- Then return to a neutral position, lying on your back, to finish. **(F)**

TOP TIP

Make sure the movement is controlled and flowing, and avoid stretching or stressing your neck muscles.

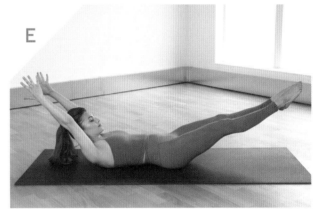

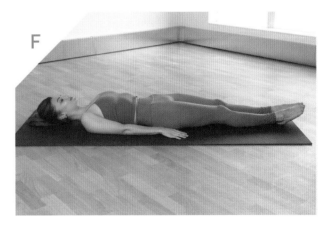

BRIDGE POSE

This core Pilates move is a wonderful stretch for the front of your body and great for strengthening the back. You're aiming for a straight line from shoulders to knees, without any arching of the back.

- Lie on your back with bent knees hip-width apart, your feet flat on the floor and your arms by your sides, palms downward. **(A)**
- Inhale as you engage your core and begin to lift your tailbone off the mat, pressing your lower spine into the mat as you raise your body so your pelvis tilts toward you. **(B)**
- Continue to peel your spine off the mat, vertebra by vertebra, until you are resting on your shoulder blades and feet. Hold the pose for 30 seconds and breathe naturally, concentrating on keeping your spine long. Then on an exhale, slowly roll your spine back down to the mat. Repeat 5–8 times, remembering to inhale as you go up and exhale when you come down. **(C)**

TOP TIP
Be sure to keep your knees in line with your hip, rather than letting them fall outward.

BRIDGE WITH DIPS VARIATION
When in the raised position, try dipping down so that your bottom is just above the floor, then rising up again. Repeat 12 times.

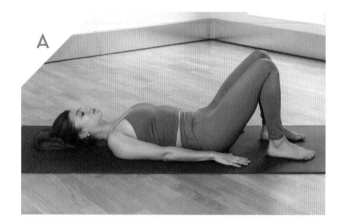

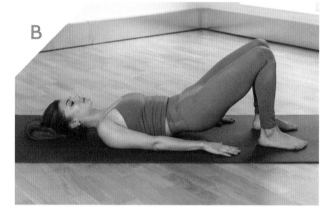

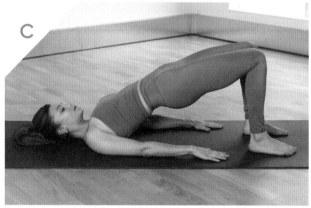

REVERSE BRIDGE WITH LEG LIFT

Like a plank, this is a fearsome move that works the core, the muscles down the back of the body and the glutes. Again, imagine a glass of water on your abdomen during this one and try to keep the water from spilling. Slow and steady wins!

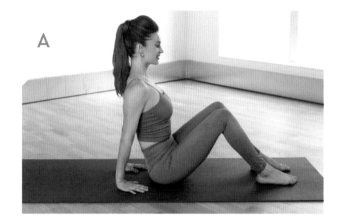

- Start in a seated position with your knees bent and your feet flat on the mat. Keep your spine straight and place your hands on the floor behind you with your fingers pointing toward your body. **(A)**
- Engage your core and inhale as you lift your bottom up into what is called a reverse bridge – where your body is in a straight, horizontal line from knees to head. **(B)**
- Once you have the position secure, exhale as you raise your right knee up at a right angle – so that your upper leg is vertical and your lower leg horizontal. **(C)**
- Do this 6 times, then do the same move 6 times with your left knee.
- To end, slowly and gently lower your bottom to the floor.

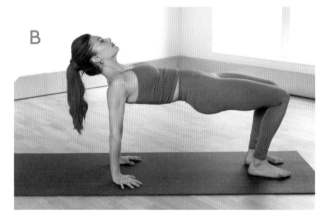

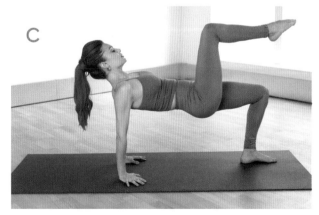

DONKEY KICKS

I love a simple backward kick from all fours – called a "donkey kick" – for getting the blood flowing! This move is particularly great for the glutes.

- Start on all fours in a tabletop position, with shoulders stacked over the wrists and knees directly beneath the hips. **(A)**
- On an exhale, kick your right leg, bent at a right angle, back and up, as high as is comfortable. **(B)**
- Repeat 10 times on the right leg and then swap sides and do the same with the left leg.

PUSH-UP VARIATION

If you want to raise your game, try adding a simple push-up movement between each donkey kick.

A

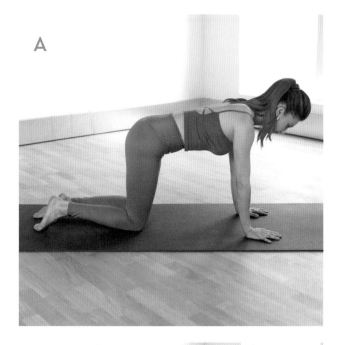

B

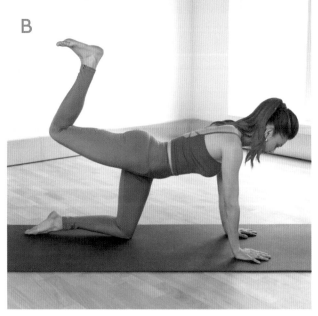

MOUNTAIN CLIMBERS

A love-or-loathe move, this one is a great all-round workout, targeting your agility, balance and co-ordination all at once. Go with speed if you'd like to get your heart rate going or go more slowly if you'd like to focus on your abs.

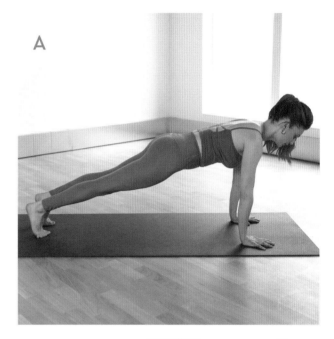

A

- Start in a high press-up position – with your bodyweight supported on hands and toes, feet hip-width apart and your body in a straight line from your shoulders down to your toes. **(A)**
- Ensuring that your arms are straight, engage your core and bend your right knee forward into a "climbing" position close to your chest, looking down to the floor in front of you as you do so. Breathe naturally throughout. **(B)**
- Return your right foot to its original position and repeat with the left knee.
- Once you are confident with the move, speed it up and keep alternating the knees for 30 seconds.

TOP TIP

When in high press-up position, be sure to keep your hands directly beneath your shoulders.

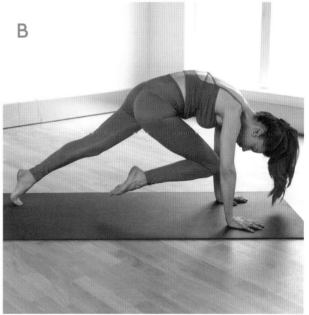

B

HIP ROLLS

This is a great move for your spine, relieving tension and challenging your core at the same time. It's particularly perfect for a day when you've spent too much time sitting down!

- Lie on your back with knees bent, your feet flat on the floor and your legs together. Extend your arms out straight at shoulder level on the floor. **(A)**
- Breathe in and engage your core and then, keeping your shoulders and upper back flat on the mat, slowly rotate your legs, still pressed together, toward the mat on the left side. Look toward the right to deepen the stretch. **(B)**
- Bring your legs carefully back to the centre and then lower them to the right this time, looking toward the left. Repeat this 5–8 times on each side.

TOP TIP
Ensure that your back doesn't arch and your shoulders stay flat and square on the mat.

LEGS RAISED VARIATION
For more of a challenge, you can perform this twisting move starting with your feet off the mat, knees bent at a right angle and lower legs parallel with the floor.

A

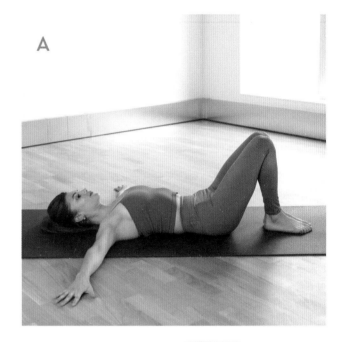

B

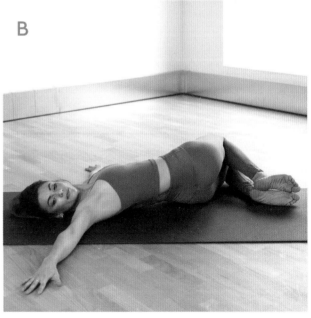

KNEES TO CHEST

This simple grounding movement is a soothing end to an exercise routine and a good stretch for the whole back and spine – a nice "hug" for the body.

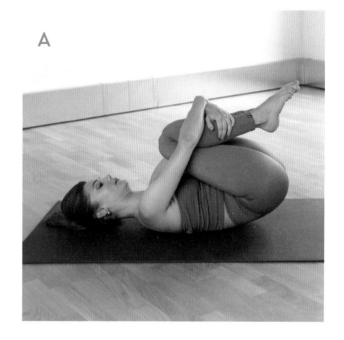

A

- Lying on your back, bring both knees up toward your chest, wrap your arms around them to hold them in position and breathe long, slow breaths for as long as you feel the need. **(A)**

TOP TIP

Never "bounce" your legs in this position and be sure to keep your hips on the floor.

STANDING VARIATION

From a standing position, hug one knee at a time up toward your chest, curling your neck forward so that your head moves toward the raised knee.

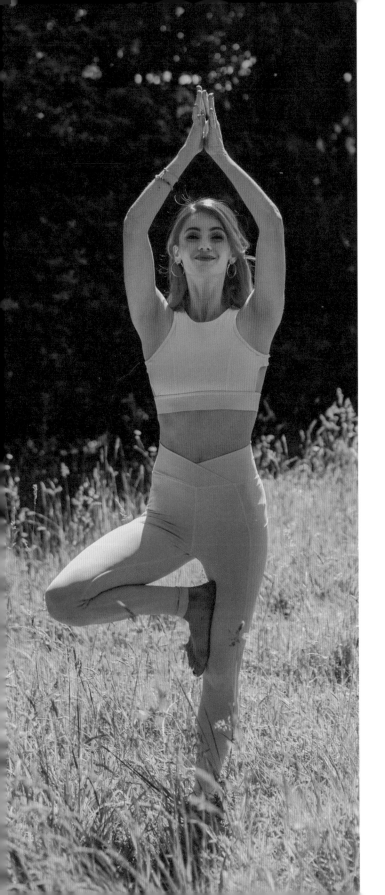

YOGA POSES TO BALANCE AND STRETCH

Yoga is something that I'm evangelical about. Whether I do it for just ten minutes or an hour, I always lose myself in my sessions. For me, it's the best way to deal with daily stress and worries, and the breath is key to this – you breathe through the poses or postures, which quietens and focuses the *mind*, while the poses themselves bring strength and flexibility to your *body*. It's just so freeing.

When I was in my late twenties, I had an unexpected break from dancing as my health was at risk. I had been dancing a minimum of four hours every day – often twice that – for eight years. So when I stopped, I struggled, as I was no longer doing the thing that gave me such joy and made me feel so good about myself – the thing that gave me such a big hit of endorphins every day. I wondered if maybe after eight years as a professional dancer, my time was up and my dancing days were over. That was when I went to my first yoga class.

At the time, hot yoga was all the rage and in Australia, where I lived, it was winter and a little cold, so I thought it might be nice to go and get warm! I saw a special offer for a month's worth of classes, so I went along and got hot and sweaty.

At first, it didn't make a lot of sense to me. But once I let myself really feel what the teachers were trying to say to me, I became totally hooked on the feeling it gave me. It was a bit like dancing again – the breathing and movement working together to simultaneously lift and ground me.

From the very first session, I was told "Don't look at anyone around the room; it's not about them, it's about your own journey." Coming from the world of dance, where you're so often looking around the room trying to dance better than the other people, that was just so refreshing and uplifting – a powerful learning curve that came at just the right time. All I needed was my mat and to move my body!

I was soon obsessed with yoga and wanted to try out more styles – something more calming and restorative too, so I tried yin yoga and breath work, among others. I loved exploring the different styles.

Yoga as Therapy

I had lost my way in life somewhat, but the yoga made my body and mind stronger and helped me feel that whatever had happened, something good was coming next. It gave me a sense of positivity when I had lost my faith in myself, lost my connection with my body and almost given up.

I have confidence as a dancer but doing yoga gave me something quite different. The minute I started, I felt completely calm and comfortable, right from the very first class. And one reason was because it didn't feel like anyone was judging me, which meant I could go at my own pace. Everyone was there for themselves, and it felt like a safe haven. I still carry that safe feeling with me even when I'm practising on my own.

Yoga encouraged me to focus more on my strengths, and to appreciate and believe in myself again – and that's when all the things I really wanted in life started to come to me. I received a great new job offer and, once I was well enough, I joined Australia's *Dancing with the Stars*, which then led to the UK and *Strictly Come Dancing*. My life had turned around!

It's amazing how, when you really notice and concentrate on the things that you can do and "own" that, the more you start to notice, and indeed grow, the positives.

What is Yoga?

I was a little intimidated to go to a yoga class at first as I expected it to be all spiritual and mystical. I'm quite a spiritual soul as it happens, but I was worried in case I wouldn't know what I was supposed to do. Would I look stupid? Would I be able to do the moves? But it turns out that I needn't have worried ...

Yoga dates back over 5,000 years to ancient India. In its simplest form, it's a mind-body practice that involves moving the body through a series of postures, or poses (called asanas) – in a "yoga flow". The poses work on the muscles, ligaments, joints and nerves in the body as well as on the mind. And different poses stimulate different parts of the physical and energetic body, releasing tension.

However, while it is indeed an ancient practice seeped in history and theory, it's also easy to learn, feels very appropriate for our modern busy way of living, and it's easy to adapt it to whatever you want from it – be it to help train a healthy body, improve mental strength or build a more spiritual way of life.

There are plenty of different styles of yoga – some more slow and calming; others more dynamic. I like trying all the styles for the different ways they make me feel, both physically and mentally, which means that I often pop into new classes when I'm travelling. Working with a variety of teachers means that I still learn something new at every yoga class!

Yogic Breathing

Breathing is as important a part of yoga as doing the physical movements, as the breath is the key to true union between body and mind.

Taking long, slow breaths as you move through yoga poses works to soothe your nervous system, effectively sending a message to your body to be calm – reassuring it that everything is well and triggering your relaxation response. With calm, regulated breathing, your heart rate, blood pressure and stress hormones, such as cortisol, will diminish, and your lungs will strengthen. According to a Sanskrit saying, "For breath is life; if you breathe well, you will live long on earth."

You might want to turn back to the more specific breathing techniques that I mentioned on pages 39–40 when you have a few minutes: Alternate Nostril Breathing, the 4–7–8 Technique and Lion's Breath. These can be used as a tool to help you feel calmer and less stressed at *any* time.

As you do the yoga poses that I outline in the pages that follow, the idea is to concentrate on trying to breathe consciously, both in *and* out through the nose, during *all* your movements, in order to provide a warmer, healthier breath for the lungs and other body systems. And you can choose to breathe more deeply into certain postures to create more length, stretch and power if desired.

It took me a while to be able to think about breathing and movement at the same time. And I'm still learning where to inhale and exhale, and how to breathe to get the most out of the postures and practices. But generally, you exhale as you bend, and you inhale as you open the front of the body.

Yoga makes me aware that my inhalations and exhalations are all coming from within. That's one of the many wonderful things about yoga – how it helps you to understand the way your own body works. To really understand this aspect of yoga is a huge and beautiful long-term gain. Like with dancing, you never stop learning when you practise yoga. I still learn something new through it every day!

When I started practising, I tended to focus on purely the physical movements. It wasn't until I spent time at a restorative yoga class and became more used to the movements that I began to understand and appreciate the breathing aspect.

I'm generally a total "go-go-go" person, so the breathing aspect allowed me to slow down enough to see how yoga nurtures both body *and* mind. Being able to consciously create moments of controlled breathing, relaxation and calm on the yoga mat helped me to be able to make the most of my more "full-on" moments both on and off the mat. And I particularly enjoyed the fact that I could control my anxiety with breathing.

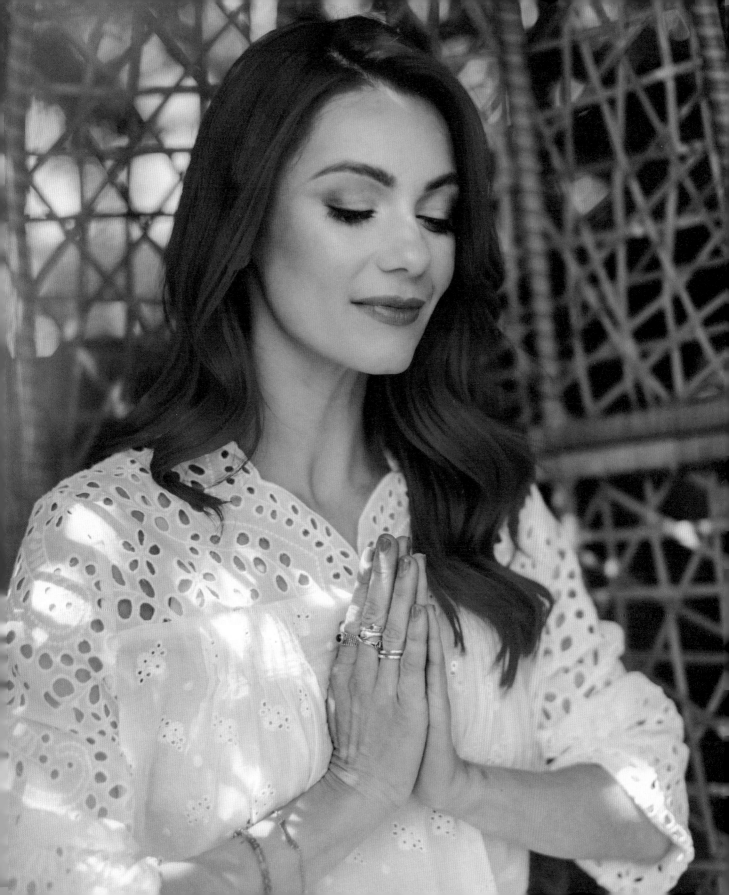

Having said all this though, I don't want you to get overly hung up on the breathing aspect when doing the poses in the pages that follow. Just try to follow the prompts within the exercise text in terms of when to inhale and exhale with the various movements. The more you practice, the easier it will get. Meanwhile, the most important thing is to keep breathing – and not hold your breath!

Other Health Benefits

Yoga is amazing for all-round wellbeing. One of the first things I noticed when I started practising it was the quite dramatic improvement in my flexibility – one of the things I often want to work on, as a dancer. I was genuinely surprised how much of a difference it made! It also had a notable effect on my muscle strength. We often tend to think of strength exercise as lifting weights, but yoga gave me the most toned muscles that I had ever gained from one form of exercise! Given that I was used to full-on exercise as a professional dancer, I really hadn't expected such amazing physical side-effects from a regular yoga practice but if you're doing it right, yoga seems to use every single muscle in your body!

Yoga is also brilliant for good quality sleep, which is so important! Even just doing a little yoga before bed can help you to wind down. There have been so many nights that I wasn't sure *why* I couldn't sleep – I just didn't feel ready or prepared for it. If I'm feeling restless at night-time these days, I do yoga for five or ten minutes max and it gets my head in a calmer, more relaxed space.

The other major upside of yoga for me was the way it helped my self-confidence and all-round mental health, especially when things felt so difficult as I wasn't able to dance. As you have to focus on both the movement and controlling the breath, you don't tend to think about other things going on. With other forms of exercise, my mind will wander as I move, but when I'm thinking about the breathing and stretching of yoga, I'm in the moment and I stress and worry less, making the session extra therapeutic. Nowadays, when I have a day on which I'm feeling a little anxious or unsure of things, yoga is the exercise I choose. And when I wake up in the morning and start the day with even just five minutes of yoga, I instantly feel loads better – like I want to conquer the world!

Equipment

It's a good idea to have a yoga mat to work on – it will cushion your joints and provide traction in your poses, making things more comfortable for you. Yoga blocks and straps can also be helpful. People don't talk about using these as much as I think they should – they support you in the poses, helping you to avoid forcing yourself into a posture if your muscles won't move far enough for correct alignment. As a dancer, I have a good understanding of my body, and also good flexibility, but if you're just starting out on your journey with movement, it's important to use blocks or straps if you're not as flexible. It's all too easy to watch Mr or Mrs Bendy in a yoga class achieving every move with ease and to then expect the same of ourselves, but the reality is that most of us could really benefit from using blocks or straps in many poses.

Such props are in no way "cheats" or signs that we "aren't flexible enough" – they're simply part of allowing *everyone* to achieve the same core moves without strain or injury. Once you try using them, you'll realize how valuable they are for many of us – so you'll see that I suggest potentially using them for certain poses in the pages that follow, although you're welcome to use them to help with any postures, of course, so feel free to look up the best ways to do so online if you'd like to explore this side of things further.

I'm so glad to share some yoga with you in this book, as a regular yoga practice has completely changed me. For someone who had movement as a major part of my day for almost my entire life, it took finding yoga to really change my relationship with exercise. Yoga taught me the invaluable lesson that positive, healthy movement is not about being better than others, or the best! It's about meeting and loving your body where it is *right now*. And it totally showed me, in an accessible way, just how intrinsically linked to movement wellbeing is for me.

Yoga really can provide huge health and wellness gains if you can find even just five or ten minutes a day for it. In fact, it has been proven that doing as little as this every day is better than doing an hour or so every week. So let's put our health first by getting familiar with the yoga poses that follow – so that they can become part of your regular daily movement practice.

YOGA POSES

1. Happy Baby
2. Cat-Cow
3. Mountain Pose
4. Standing Forward Fold
5. Tree Pose
6. Halfway Lift
7. Downward Dog
8. One-legged Dog
9. Upward Dog
10. Chaturanga (Low Plank)
11. Wild Thing
12. Lizard Lunge
13. Half Pigeon
14. Warrior 1
15. Warrior 2
16. Warrior 3
17. Triangle Pose
18. Chair Pose
19. Puppy Pose
20. Child's Pose

"Yoga really can provide huge health and wellness gains if you can find even just five or ten minutes a day for it."

HAPPY BABY

I often do this pose after I've been dancing for a long time and my hips tighten up – especially if I've been wearing dancing shoes! It always makes me smile.

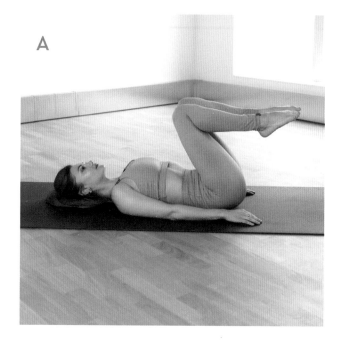

A

- Start by lying flat on your back on the mat. Then on an exhale, bring your knees slowly toward your chest. (A)
- Next, allow your legs to fall outward. Flex your feet and reach up to take hold of a foot in each hand, keeping your shoulders, neck and head on the floor. Rock gently from side to side on your back for a minute, like a "happy baby", breathing slowly and deeply as you do so. (B)

TOP TIP

The soles of your feet should be flat, as if you are trying to walk on the ceiling.

EASIER VARIATION

If your hands don't reach your feet, you can use yoga straps to bridge the gap, or hold on to your shins or ankles instead of your feet. (With my tight hips, I still have to use a band to reach the posture I want.)

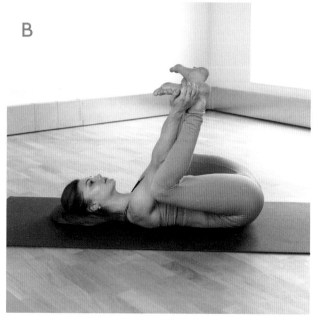

B

CAT-COW

Cat–Cow is one of my favourite yoga moves. It's easy and highly beneficial, especially if you need a little posture corrector after you've been sitting at a desk all day.

- Start on all fours in a tabletop position, with your shoulders directly above your wrists, and your hips directly above your knees. Your fingertips should be facing forward, and ensure that you maintain a neutral spine. Keep your head and neck in line with your back rather than looking up or down. **(A)**
- To move into Cow pose, inhale and engage your abdominal muscles, then tilt your tailbone backward and upward, drop your stomach, feeling your spine stretch, and lift your head gently so you are looking up. **(B)**
- To move into Cat pose, exhale and tuck under your tailbone, moving from your pelvis and letting your spine arch upward. Feel the rounding of your spine as you tuck your head under. **(C)**
- Repeat the Cow-Cat sequence 8–10 times, being sure to marry each movement with the breath. Finish in a neutral spine position.

TOP TIP
Lead the movements from your tailbone, rather than with your head or neck.

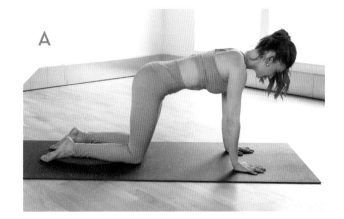

A

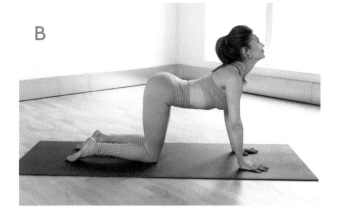

B

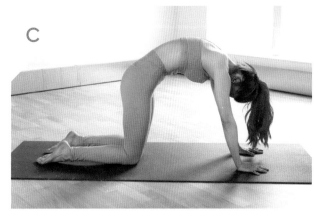

C

MOUNTAIN POSE

The foundation for most other standing poses, this move looks simple but is deceptively powerful in terms of its ability to increase your awareness of healthy body alignment.

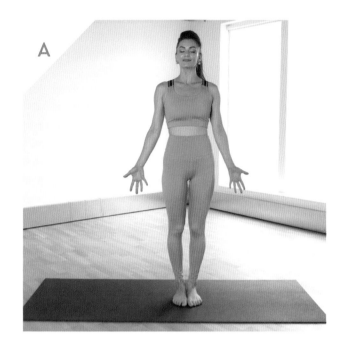

A

- Stand tall with your feet together and firmly rooted to the floor, your arms by your side, palms facing forward, and your core engaged. Concentrate on your body's alignment, stacking your rib cage on top of your hips and keeping your legs straight but with soft knees. Engage your quadriceps (the muscles on the front of your thighs) to lift your kneecaps. Ensure that your shoulders are down and away from your ears, drawn backward toward your spine. Breathe gently as you hold this position for 3–5 breaths. (A)

TOP TIP
Concentrate on elongating your body and feeling all your muscles working to anchor the position. And smile – our face is the first place where we hold tension!

STANDING FORWARD FOLD

This lovely forward fold is such a great all-rounder for lengthening muscles, relieving tension and working on your posture. Enjoy the stretch that it creates right up and down your body.

- Stand tall with your feet about hip-width apart, reach your arms toward the ceiling, inhale and engage your core. **(A)**
- With your knees slightly soft, slowly fold your body forward on an exhale. Start by tucking in your chin. Next, round your upper chest, then allow your back to fold down one vertebra at a time until your hands are as close to the floor as possible. Only bend over as far as is comfortable – and hold for a full breath there. **(B)**
- Then, with your core still firmly engaged, inhale and slowly roll your body back up to standing, from the bottom vertebra upward. Your head should be the last part of you to come up.

TOP TIP

Ensure that your shoulders are down and away from your ears at both the beginning and end of this pose.

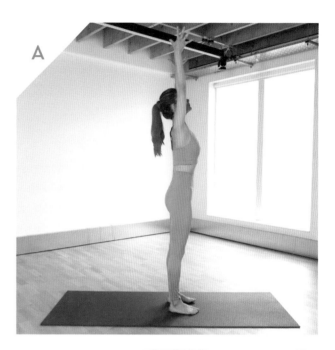

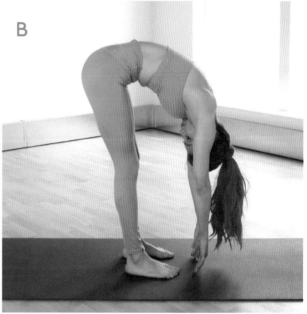

TREE POSE

A favourite yoga move of many, this graceful balancing pose, inspired by the steady but flexible grace of trees, often follows on from Mountain Pose.

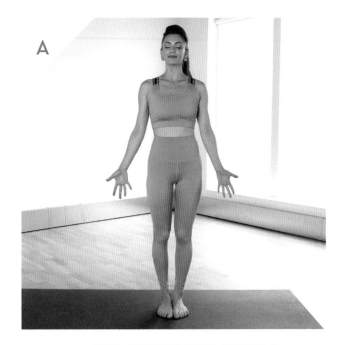

A

- Start in Mountain Pose (see page 126 for more guidance), or simply standing upright with your feet together. (A)
- Draw your right foot up to sit against your left inner thigh, with your toes pointing down your leg. Then raise your hands together in prayer position firstly at chest level and, if you're steady there, then above your head. Hold the pose for 3–5 breaths, or as long as you are comfortable. (B)
- Then slowly come back to standing tall on both feet with your arms by your sides before repeating the pose on your other leg.

TOP TIP
Try and lift out of the hip of your standing leg so as not to put all your weight on one side.

EASIER VARIATION
Use your hand, or a yoga strap, to keep your raised foot in place if it helps, or instead put your foot on your lower leg. Or you could try this pose standing with your back against a wall, or even holding the wall for support if required.

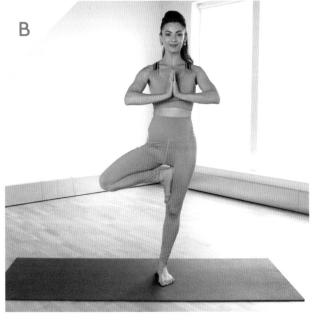

B

HALFWAY LIFT

This pose is useful to learn as it often links other standing yoga poses as part of a flowing yoga sequence. Be sure that you do it with a straight back, not a curved one.

- Start in either Mountain Pose, with your arms raised above your head, or in Standing Forward Fold – see page 126 and 127 for more guidance. **(A) (B)**
- On an inhale, either lower or lift your upper body halfway up with a flat back into a horizontal back position, holding your legs lightly with your arms and keeping your core muscles engaged. Hold this for 1 breath. **(C)**
- Then, on an exhale, move through to your next position.

TOP TIP

Keep your knees soft (i.e. ever so slightly bent) rather than locked, and remember to focus on the breath as you move into position.

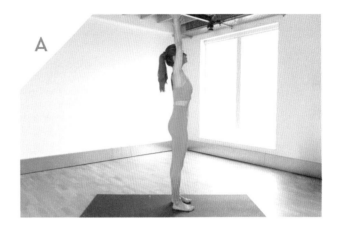

A

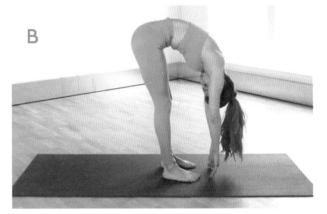

B

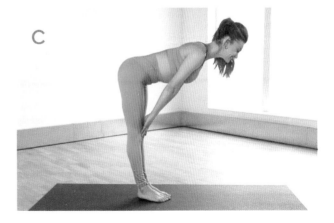

C

DOWNWARD DOG

I rarely do a yoga sequence that doesn't include a Downward Dog. This all-time favourite pose of mine stretches your back, arms, hamstrings, front of legs ... The list goes on, as I feel it covers everything, plus it's a great grounding pose as well.

- Start on all fours in a tabletop position, with your knees directly under your hips, your wrists directly under your shoulders, your fingers facing forward and the tops of your toes touching the floor. (A)
- Then tuck your toes under and, on an exhale, lift your knees up from the floor and your tailbone up toward the ceiling, feeling yourself rise from your core and hips, rather than pushing yourself into position with your hands. Keep your legs slightly bent at this point and be sure to root the palm of your hands firmly into the floor. (B)

A

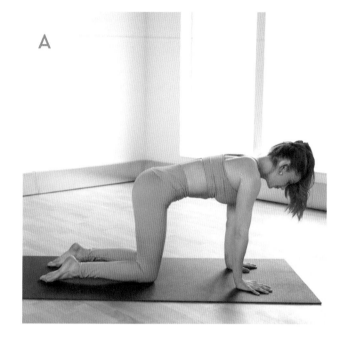

B

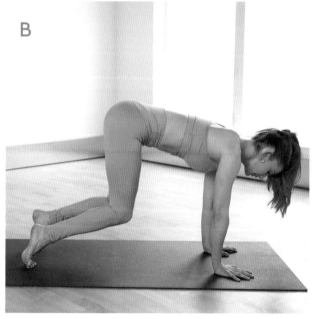

- Hold for 1 breath, then exhale and push backward with the top of your thighs to straighten your legs as much as you can, without locking your knees. Aim to get your heels onto the floor – but this is hard, so just be aware that you may not be able to do it straight away! Hold the pose for 5 breaths. **(C)**
- Then, on the next exhale, bend your knees and return to all fours on the mat.

TOP TIP

Make sure that your shoulder blades are wide and pulling down your back, rather than moving up toward your ears.

TWIST VARIATION

While in full Downward Dog (final step), reach one arm toward your leg on the opposite side while keeping your hips and legs still. Hold for a full breath. Repeat with the other arm.

C

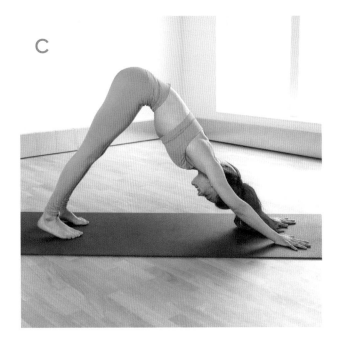

ONE-LEGGED DOG

A variation of the standard Downward Dog, this is a great way to add a balance element to this energizing pose. Be sure to keep your pelvis still as you raise your leg.

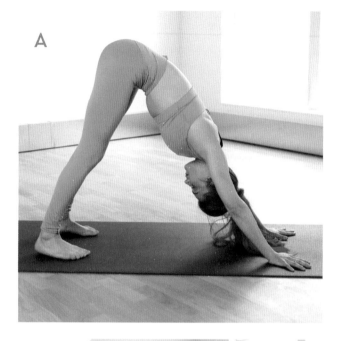

- Start in Downward Dog – see pages 130–1 for more guidance. **(A)**
- Then, on an exhale, lift your right leg up behind you so that it is in line with your torso, being careful to keep your hips still as you do so. Hold for 1 breath. **(B)**
- Then repeat the same thing with your left leg.

KNEE TO ELBOW VARIATION
While in the position, bring the knee of your raised leg down toward the opposite elbow and return.

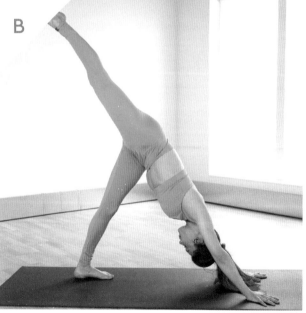

UPWARD DOG

This pose provides a wonderful back and abdominal extension with a great strengthening action for your arms and chest.

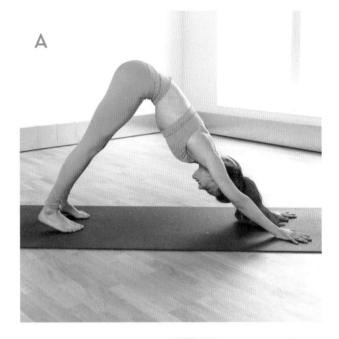

- Start in Downward Dog – see pages 130–1 for more guidance. (A)
- Then, on an inhale, push your hips forward and right down toward the mat (without them touching it), allowing your head, shoulders and chest to move upward and away from the mat – so that your body ends up in a nice, curved shape, securely balanced on only your hands and the top of your feet. Keep your elbows close to your body, straighten your arms and ensure that your shoulder blades are pulling down, away from your ears. Hold this position for 1 breath. (B)
- Then, on the next exhale, gently lower yourself to the floor.

TOP TIP
Be sure to root your arms and hands firmly into the mat to keep yourself steady in this position.

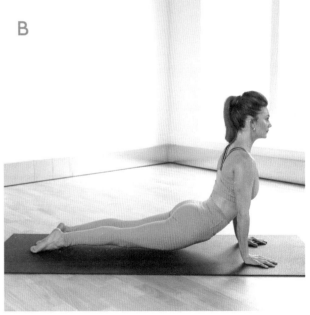

CHATURANGA (LOW PLANK)

Along with Downward Dog, this pose is a pivotal transitional position in a yoga flow sequence, often leading into an Upward Dog.

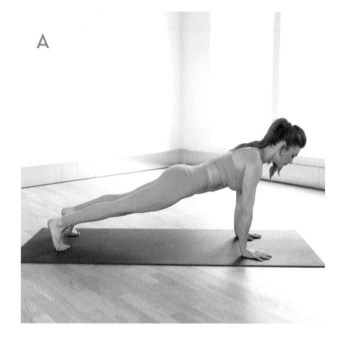

- Start in a standard Plank position – balancing on your hands and toes, with your arms straight, and your body in a straight line from head to toe. (A)
- Making sure your core is engaged, shift your upper body forward so that your shoulders move beyond your wrists. Then, on an exhale, bend your elbows so that you lower toward the floor in a controlled way until your shoulders are as much in line with your elbows as possible. Hold this for a full breath, or longer if you want. (B)
- Then, on an inhale, flow through to the next pose in a sequence or gently lower to the floor.

TOP TIP

Keep your elbows close to your body for maximum support, and use your back and core muscles to hold the position.

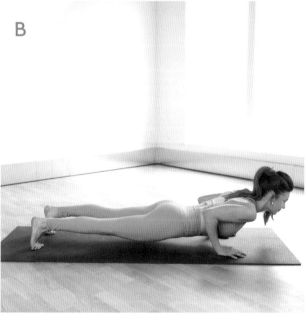

WILD THING

This dynamic pose – which is a little more "dance-y" than much of the other yoga in this book – requires both strength and flexibility but be a bit "wild" and give it a go.

- Begin seated on the floor with your right knee bent, your right foot on the mat, your left leg straight out in front of you and your left hand flat on the floor behind you, palm down, fingers facing back. **(A)**
- On an inhale, press off your right foot to lift your body so you come up into your left hand and left foot – your left leg will turn outward as you do so, opening up your hip. Come up onto the toes of your right foot and push them against the mat to help you balance, holding your right arm above you to keep yourself steady. Push down with your left hand to hold the pose, ensuring that your shoulders are not hunching up to your neck. Hold this for 3–5 breaths. **(B)**
- Then, on an exhale, slowly come back down to a seated position before switching legs and doing the pose on the other side.

A

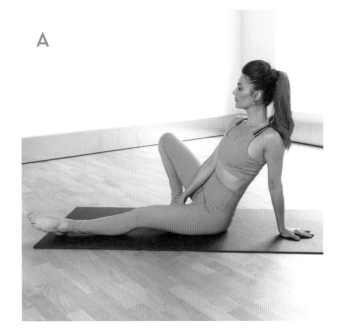

B

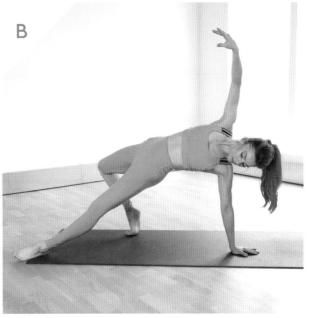

LIZARD LUNGE

This pose is an amazing opener for the hips, and one that I often do before I dance. I can stay in it for ages, but I sometimes use a block. Placing a block under your hands or elbows will help you to ease a little more into the posture.

- Start in Downward Dog – see page 130–1 for more guidance. **(A)**
- Then, on an exhale, bring your left foot forward so that it is flat on the mat, turning slightly outward, on the outside of your left hand, and your left knee is bent at a right angle, directly above your ankle. Hold this position for 5 breaths, ensuring a straight line from the top of your head down to your right ankle, and anchoring your right heel toward the mat for stability. **(B)**
- On the next inhale, step backward with your left leg and peel up into Downward Dog before repeating Step 1 on the other side.

ARM VARIATION

To add a rotation to this move, reach your right arm toward the ceiling and backward, letting your right shoulder move with it and opening the chest area. Hold for a breath, then bring your arm back to the mat.

A

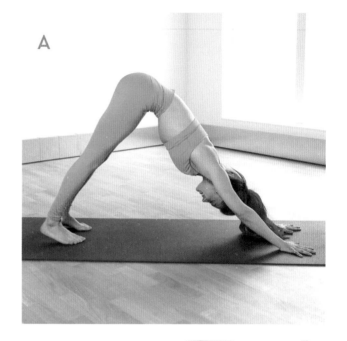

B

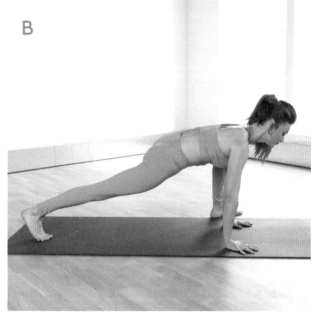

HALF PIGEON

This is a great cool-down stretch when you've been working hard on your lower body. If you are new to the pose or want to be able to ease into it, you can add a block under the buttock of your bent leg.

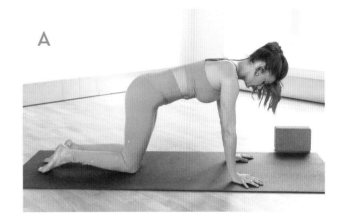

A

- Start on all fours, in a tabletop position, with your shoulders directly above your wrists and your hips directly above your knees. **(A)**

- On an inhale, move your weight forward and bring your right knee toward your right wrist. Place both your knee and shin on the mat so that your front foot sits in a comfortable position toward your groin. Slide your left leg back along the mat and point your left toes. Feel free to place the block beneath your right buttock if you feel it would be useful at any point for either support and/or alignment. **(B)**

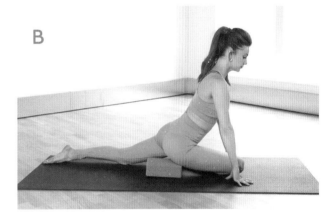

B

- Once you are comfortable, walk your hands forward as far as you can. Then, on an inhale, lift your rib cage and open your chest and, on the next exhale, lower your upper body as far as you can toward the mat. Rest your forearms and forehead on the mat if you can. Hold this position for 5 breaths. **(C)**

- To come out of the pose, push back through your hands on an exhale, lift your hips and return to tabletop position. Then repeat with your left leg forward and your right leg extended behind.

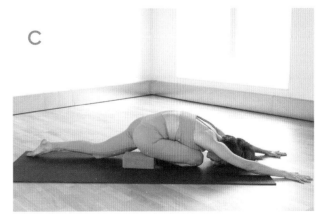

C

WARRIOR 1

I love the three Warrior poses – they give such a sense of power. They each have distinctive leg and foot alignments but are amazing whole-body yoga experiences. In this, the first of them, the hips are facing forward over the bent knee, and your arms are raised high.

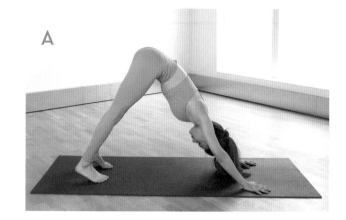

- Start in Downward Dog – see page 130–1. (A)
- Then, on an exhale, step your left foot forward in line with your right hand, allowing your back (right) foot to come up onto the toes, and bend your front (left) knee to a right-angle lunge – so that your upper thigh is parallel to the floor, with your knee directly over your ankle. (B)

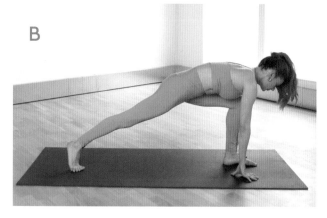

- Now, on an exhale, turn your back (right) heel inward so that your foot is flat on the floor, with your toes turned out at a 45-degree angle toward the right edge of the mat, and your heels are roughly in line with one another. Straighten your body to upright while reaching your hands straight above you, shoulder-width apart, with your palms facing each other. Separate your shoulder blades and hold for 5 breaths. (C)
- To come out of the pose, release your hands back to the floor and return to your Downward Dog position.
- Repeat the whole move on the other side, lunging forward with your right leg this time.

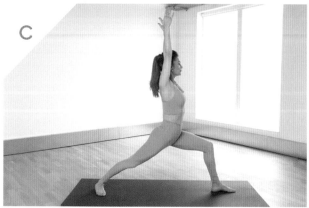

WARRIOR 2

Warrior 2 can be done either by stepping into it from a standing position or straight from Warrior 1. Your hips and upper body both face the side of the mat, and your arms are out wide, giving you a strong stretch along the side of your body.

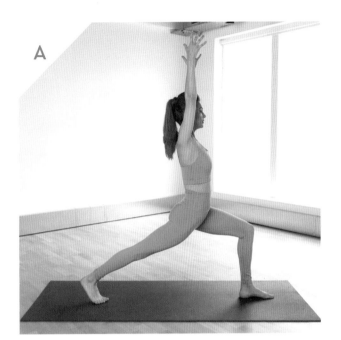

- From standing, step your left leg out in front of you, on an exhale, into a high lunge, with your body upright and your arms raised straight above you. Your left knee should be at a right-angle, your knee stacked over your ankle and the heel of your back foot raised off the floor. **(A)**

- Turn your back (right) heel inward so that your foot is flat on the floor, with your toes turned out toward the right edge of the mat. Then, on an inhale, bring your arms out to the sides at shoulder height. On an exhale, turn your upper body to face the side of the mat. Look forward beyond your left hand. Then adjust your position to feel steady – your weight should be evenly distributed between both legs, with your shoulders and rib cage stacked over your hips. Press down through the outer edge of your back foot for stability. Hold for 5 breaths. **(B)**

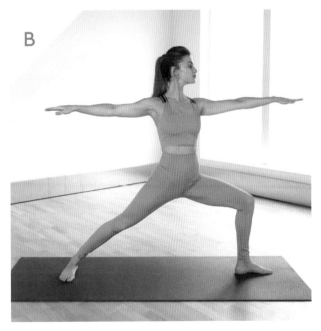

- To come out of the pose, straighten your front leg and lower your arms.

- Repeat the whole move on the other side, lunging onto your right leg this time.

WARRIOR 3

Warrior 3 is a fun but challenging balancing pose that requires a lot of focus to hold your body in a "T" shape – with one leg out behind you, your body as parallel to the floor as you can get it and your arms out wide in line with your shoulders.

- From standing, step your left leg out in front of you and, on an exhale, move into a high lunge, with your body upright and your arms raised straight above you. **(A)**
- Slowly lean forward to transfer your body weight onto your front leg. And, on an inhale, lower your torso until it is parallel with the floor, straighten your front (left) leg and lift your back (right) leg straight out behind you, keeping your arms down by your sides. **(B)**

A

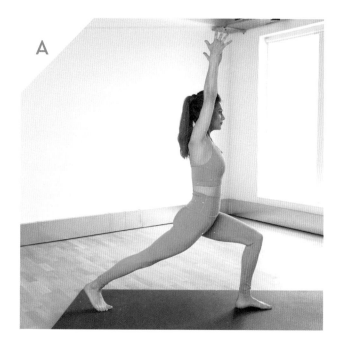

B

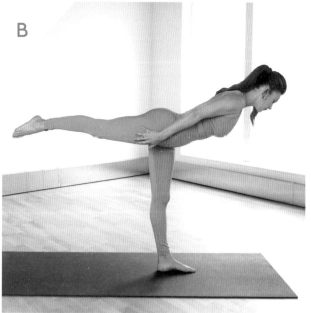

- Take a few breaths in this position and, when you feel stable, on an inhale, move your arms out to the sides at shoulder height – so that they are parallel with the floor and your whole body forms a "T" shape. Hold for 3–5 breaths. (C)
- To come out of the pose, return your back foot to the floor behind you and rise back up to your high lunge position.
- Switch legs and repeat the move on the other side, putting your body weight forward onto your right leg this time.

TOP TIP

Take your time on these moves – they are very uplifting and powerful when done properly.

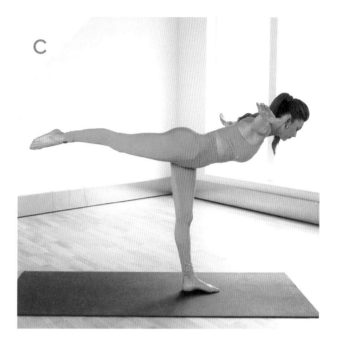

C

TRIANGLE POSE

The Triangle Pose is great to help you improve body alignment awareness as you look directly up at your hand to get that lovely triangle shape with your body. Don't worry if you can't get your hand the whole way down to the floor – you can always use a block to bridge the gap.

- From standing with your feet a comfortable width apart, turn to face the side of the mat, engage your core and move your feet to a wide stance – wider than shoulder-width. Then stretch your arms directly outward, level with your shoulders, and turn your left foot out to follow the direction of your left arm. **(A)**
- Next, shift your hips toward the back of the mat and, on the next inhale, reach as far forward as you can from the waist, keeping your spine long and straight. **(B)**

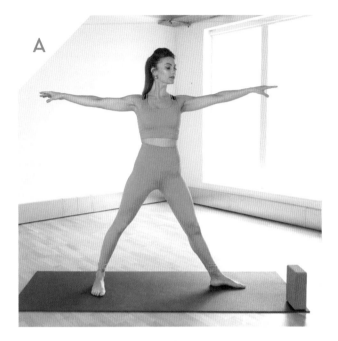

A

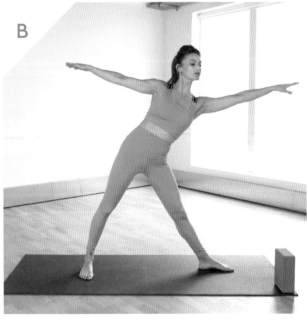

B

- On an exhale, lower your left arm down toward the mat, aiming to place your left fingertips on the mat inside of your left foot. Don't worry if you can't reach this far though – you can simply either hold your left leg higher up or place a block on the floor for you to lower your hand onto. Once comfortable here, raise your right arm straight up in the air, with the palm of your hand facing forward, and look up toward your right hand. Hold the pose for 3–5 breaths. **(C) (D)**
- Then, on an inhale, slowly return to standing and repeat the whole move on the other side, starting by turning your right foot out to follow the direction of your right arm.

TOP TIP

Keep your legs straight when reaching for the floor, but without locking your knee joints.

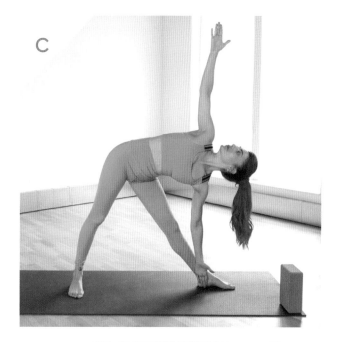

C

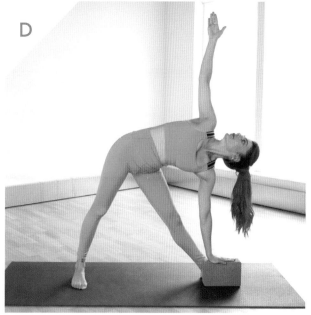

D

CHAIR POSE

This deceptively challenging but strengthening pose is one to practise with the long-term in mind. Take it steady and work on the technique before aiming for long holds.

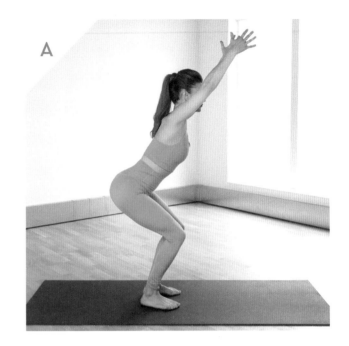

A

- Stand with your feet hip-width apart. On an inhale, bend your knees into a deep squat, as if you are sitting into a chair, and raise your arms above your head, just in front of your ears, with your palms facing inward. Due to the sitting action, your bottom should be directed downward and slightly backward, while your upper body should be leaning slightly forward, so that it forms a rough right angle with the tops of your thighs. Ensuring that your core is engaged, your thighs are parallel to one another and your spine is long, hold the pose for 3–5 breaths, breathing deeply here. With practice, you should be able to hold the pose for longer. (A)

CALF RAISE VARIATION
Rise up onto your toes while in the "seated" position, then come back to flat feet again.

PUPPY POSE

This is a deeply soothing, restorative position for the upper back and shoulders. My shoulders tend to get sore from holding my arms up so much of the time when dancing, so this move feels particularly great for me. I also love the stretch I get in my hips when I settle into it.

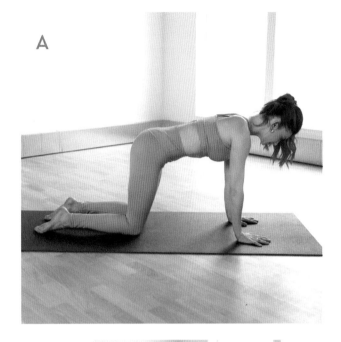

- Start on all fours in a tabletop position, with your shoulders directly above your hands, your hips directly above your knees and the tops of your feet flat against the floor. **(A)**
- Then walk your hands forward and, on an exhale, lower your chest toward the floor while leaving your hips in the air. Aim to place your forehead on the mat if you can, and feel your spine stretch, keeping a natural curve in your lower back and your thighs at right angles to the floor. **(B)**

TOP TIP
Keep your feet in line with your hips, and your hips square as you lengthen your spine.

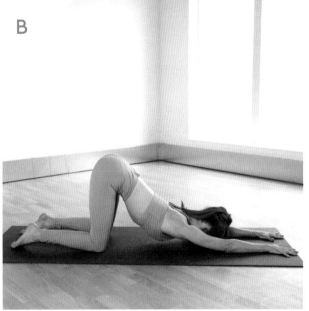

CHILD'S POSE

The Child's Pose is an amazing tension reliever, an instant posture corrector and a common counter-pose for many back stretches, such as Downward Dog. It lengthens and stretches not just your back, shoulders and neck area, but also your thighs and ankles.

- Start on all fours in a tabletop position, with your shoulders directly above your hands, your hips directly above your knees and the tops of your feet flat against the floor. **(A)**
- On an exhale, sit back, bringing your bottom toward your ankles, and reach your arms along the mat in front of you, flattening your body as far toward the mat as you can. If possible, rest your forehead on the mat. Breathe naturally. **(B)**

A

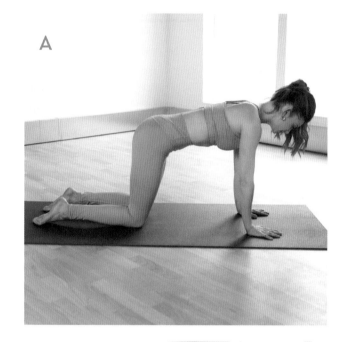

B

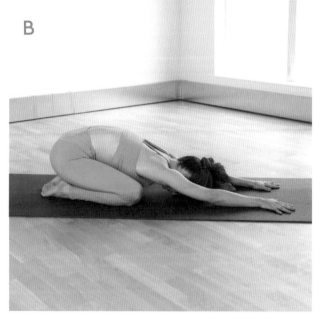

- Next, inch the fingers of both hands together slowly over to the right, feeling the move pull down the left side of your body. Then move your arms back to the centre and over to the left. Return to the centre position. **(C) (D)**

TOP TIP

To deepen the stretch, widen the position of your knees a little, keeping your feet together.

RAISED ARM VARIATION

From the centre position, lift your left arm toward the ceiling and look up at your raised hand. Return to centre and repeat with the right arm.

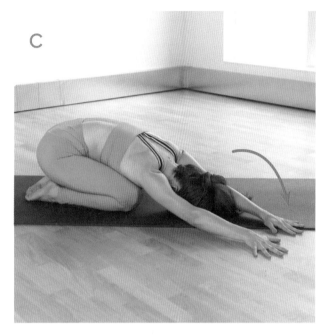

C

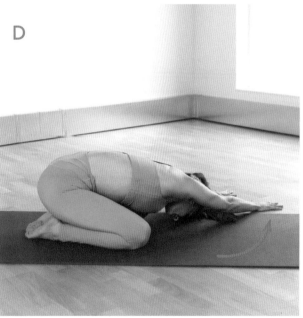

D

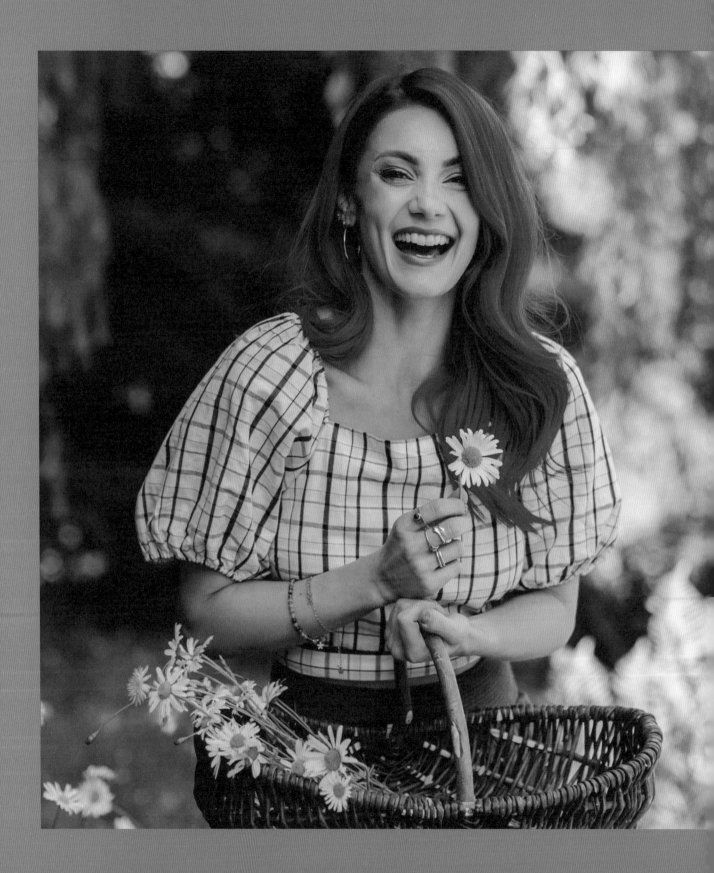

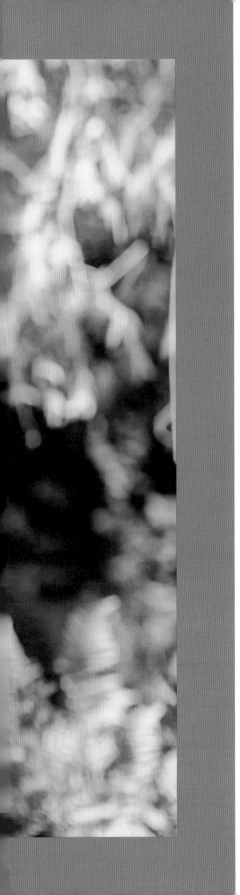

Part 3

21 Days to a Stronger, Happier You

Woohoo! This is the really fun part of the book – we're going to put all the talk into action, try out lots of different yoga, Pilates and dance routines, and find out what our bodies are capable of. The routines you'll try out over these next three weeks range from easy and short stretch routines to more challenging cardio workouts, from stretch yoga to sculpt and tone to energizing tap and salsa. The important thing is to find the enjoyment in the movement – and don't give up if the day's routine really isn't for you. This is about getting your body moving with a smile on your face. We've got something for everyone, whether you've always wanted to chassé across the *Strictly* dance floor, try a barre class, have a go at some calming yoga or strengthen your core with Pilates. Let's get moving!

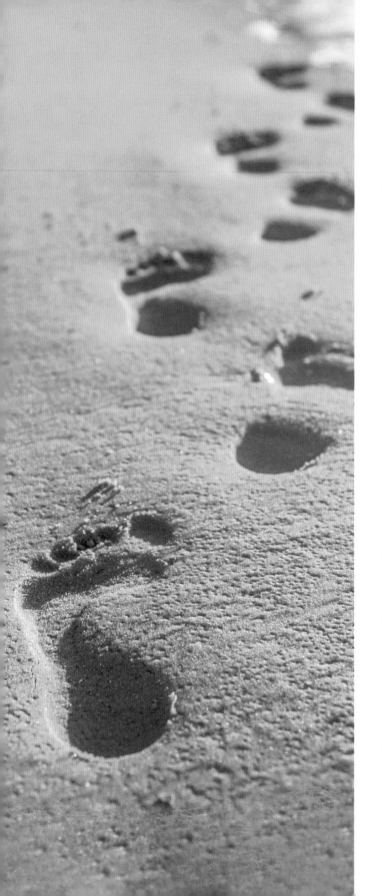

HOW TO USE THE PLAN

The Move Yourself Happy Plan is all about finding your happy place with exercise and feeling the benefits of improved strength, flexibility and energy. Simply making movement a lifestyle choice and part of your everyday routine is going to make a huge difference to how you feel. And finding a little more time to put yourself first is a bonus.

21 Days of Finding Fun in Joyful Movement

On the following pages is the Move Yourself Happy Plan – a 21-day plan that encourages you to try out different exercise routines to get your body moving more. It also includes some hacks and easy wins that embrace the principles of the Four Pillars in Part 1 (see pages 12–47). It's about putting yourself first and centre in your life and finding your way to a healthier and happier you.

On each day of the three-week plan, I've devised a routine based on yoga, Pilates or dance – or a fusion of these – using the movements from Part 2 of the book (see pages 49–147). There are restorative and calming routines, upbeat full-on days and plenty in between. The aim is to try out these different styles of movement to find out what you enjoy and what makes your body feel good.

Try not to miss a day – sometimes exercise is just the thing we need to find time for when a day is busy and tough. Carving out that five minutes for a few stretches that will help you stand tall and feel strong will improve the toughest of days.

It's easy to tell yourself "I'm not a yoga person" or think you've tried something once and it didn't do anything for you, but you never know what might click with you when you get into the rhythm of regular movement. And mixing up your exercise gives you different movement styles to choose from – so there's always a way to bring movement into your day, whatever your energy level or mood.

Nothing should take longer than 15 minutes, and most routines will take far less than this. Of course, you can always add in extra reps or do a routine twice a day if you enjoy it and have the time. And enjoyment is the key – I want you to move your body in different ways without any pressure. This is about trialing clever movements that strengthen and energize your body quickly. Here's what we're going to be doing over the next 21 days:

- Tap
- Dancer's Contemporary Flow
- Inspired Jive
- Salsa
- Arms and Abs
- Stretch Yoga
- Dancer's Tone
- Earthing Energy Booster
- Legs and Core Supersets
- Burner Cardio
- Sculpt and Tone Pilates
- Yoga For Stress Relief
- Pilates Ballet Fit
- Yoga For Balance
- Yoga and Pilates Fusion
- Heart Opener Yoga
- Hip Opener
- Power Pilates
- Awakening Flow
- Rest Day Restorative Yoga
- Short Sun Salutation

Your 21 Days

The 21 Days are broken down into three weeks – **Week 1** starts with gaining an **Awareness** of your relationship with movement and exercise, finding out what you like and trying out new healthy tools in your life. The main objective here is for you to find joy in moving your body because you want to rather than because you have to. Explore new opportunities for simple changes that help you find the joy in moving your body and nourishing both your body and mind. **Week 2** is about **Routine** – looking for patterns and ideas that will help you embed new movement habits and healthy living tools into your everyday, so that you can choose what to weave into your life going forward. You'll also try more movement routines that show you just how much fun it can be to add a little salsa, Power Pilates or restorative yoga to your week. **Week 3** is about planning for the future and setting **Movement Goals** for permanent change. You'll look at all the habits you've formed with moving more and eating better and explore how these small actions come together for big change.

None of this is supposed to be difficult, but you do need to challenge yourself to put in the effort and to consistently find some time in your day to enjoy your body.

Easy Wins For Getting Movement Into the Day

This plan will help you find those easy wins for bringing movement and healthy extras into the day. During the three weeks, we'll look at motivational tools and methods to help you make it a permanent change. Remember that slow and steady will get you to the finish line – making major change is simpler than you expect if you work with small steps and tweaks to your daily routine.

There's also a mantra and journaling point for each week, which will help you to understand more about your feelings around exercise. These will also motivate you to make better nourishment choices in your day-to-day life, as well as helping you to foster a more positive mindset.

Keep Going

You might ache! After Covid and having so much time off, I went straight back full steam ahead into *Strictly* again. Returning after every break is quite intimidating and I always think, "I hope my body remembers what to do." And it does! My body goes into muscle memory, but I'm usually sore for about the first two to three weeks, then it remembers that this is how I normally work. This will probably happen to you too – but the more regularly you exercise, the quicker your body will adapt.

When I'm teaching someone, I reassure them that their body has limits. Whether you're running a race, at the gym or dancing, you're using lots of muscles in your body, and you're also using your brain a lot, so you get physically, mentally and emotionally drained. You need to allow for the necessary rest to get the most out of the experience. I had to learn that if you keep pushing and pushing, it's not beneficial. You'll get far more out of the plan if you prioritize your rest – I've included some gentle stretch days to help you incorporate rest into your schedule.

Warming Up and Cooling Down

I always start each routine with some sort of warm-up and light stretching – to get your body moving and improve flexibility. I also give you a cool-down move, as proper cooling down is just as important as warming up.

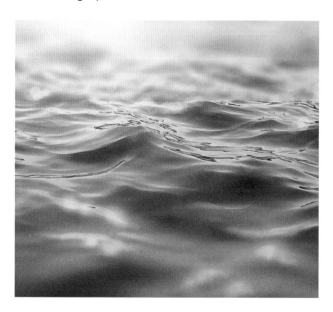

Tracking Your Progress

I'm not going to ask you to keep a record of your side plank reps, or how many minutes and seconds you've worked out each day – unless you want to. But I do want you to think about how you feel when you fit in your daily movement. How does it feel when you dance or move or work out?

The plan is all about changing your relationship with exercise and movement and how it should bring you joy, so I've created a "How Do I Feel?" tracker to help you to see how moving more makes you happier in body and mind. Each day of the plan consider the following questions and note the answers, perhaps using a scale of 1 to 10 to measure how you feel:

HOW DO YOU FEEL?

- What activities did you do today and when?
- How much energy did you have before you began your workout?
- How much energy did you feel you had after your workout?
- Did you feel that you moved enough today?
- Did the workout help your mood?

Use this like a diary for the plan to keep track of how each day or routine is making you feel. There will be good days and bad days, so this will help you to understand what works best for you and how to make exercise part of your life. Looking back at when you weren't doing this stuff and how you felt, compared to when you are doing it and how much better you're feeling, is the magic to keeping it going.

Shall We Start?

You don't need any equipment to do any of the routines. If you want to add weights to the exercises to make them more challenging then use some dumbbells or water bottles filled with rice. You might also like to use props in the yoga routines, like yoga blocks, to make some moves a bit easier.

Before you perform the exercise routine:

- Remember to warm up (and cool down afterwards).
- Why not try a simple breathing exercise (see pages 39–40)?
- Find the joy to move – put on some great music and look forward to energizing your body. Think of the movement as a treat for yourself, an indulgence to prioritize yourself, and it will help you achieve your goals.
- Think about how you feel before and afterwards – use the tracker to see how your mood improves with exercise.

"The journey of a thousand miles begins with one step."

Lao Tzu

Week 1

Awareness & Joy

MANTRA

I am. I can. I will.

DAY 1

Dancer's Tone

This is a lovely routine to start with and shows you the power of slow movement. When I'm dancing, I need a lot of strength to do the fast movements, but the slow dance moves require so much more control, which comes from the strength in your core. Regular toning exercise allows me to be able to dance like I do.

Warm-up: Side Lunges x 10 on each side

- Plié Squat with "Serving Food" Arms x 4
- Double Leg Calf Raise x 8 on each side
- Single Leg Calf Raise x 4 on each side
- First to Second Position Squat Jumps x 8
- Curtsy Squats x 4 on each side
- Plié Squat – hold for 10 seconds then pulse x 8, then repeat
- Standing Leg Lifts x 4 to front, 4 to side, 4 to back, on each side
- Mountain Pose for 3–5 breaths

Cool down: Standing Forward Fold into a Ragdoll for 5 breaths, or however long feels good

Just Move

Over these next 21 days, I want to transform your thoughts about moving your body and getting active. So many people see movement purely as an exercise thing to endure, or tell themselves they have to exercise to burn off what they've just eaten. You need to focus on having a strong body that helps you live your best life, and the amazing feelings of euphoria you get when you exercise – however you move your body. I want you to learn all about how, when you're moving more, you feel so alive and have the energy to do so much with your day. It's also about ensuring that you're putting your own health and happiness at the top of your list of must-haves in your day. Focus on those points rather than burning calories or making your body look a certain way – you're doing this just for you.

Enjoy Your Food

What are your favourite natural foods and tastes? What do you like to eat? What foods make you feel good? Do you experiment with new tastes or prefer dishes you know you like? Over the next three weeks, we're going to look at some quick and fun ways to take your nutrition up a level. At the end, I want your fridge and cupboards to be full of inspiring foods that help your body get active and feel good. We're all unique – and we all need different foods to make our bodies work at their best. Start today thinking about what you want to eat and cook more of over these next three weeks. Let's get excited about nourishing your body with good food.

Mantras

On the opening page for each week, we'll include a mantra or affirmation for you to work with. Or create your own! Write down the mantra and put it somewhere you can see it every day. Or you could repeat it every morning as an intention for your day. It's both a meditation tool and a way to reinforce your aims and encourage a positive mindset about all that you intend to achieve this week.

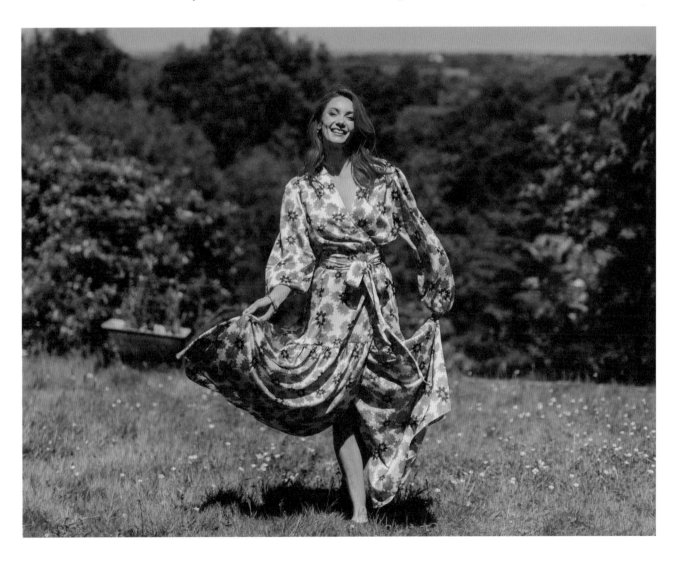

DAY 2

Yoga and Pilates Fusion

We've talked about the similarities and differences between yoga and Pilates, and what they can do for your body. I love combining them to max out my exercise time and work on my flexibility, balance and body strength all at the same time.

Warm-up: Child's Pose for 8–10 breaths

- Straight Arm Plank for 1 breath
- Mountain Climbers x 30
- Tabletop Arms and Legs x 8 on each side
- Straight Arm Plank for 1 breath
- Side Plank with Lifting Leg Variation x 6 on each side
- Straight Arm Plank for 1 breath
- Downward Dog for 3–5 breaths
- One-legged Dog with Knee to Elbow Variation x 4 on each side
- Downward Dog with Twist Variation x 4 on each side
- Repeat the routine as needed

Cool down: Child's Pose for 8–10 breaths, or however long feels good

Movement Stars

Today I want you to think about the people who you love to watch move. It could be a dancer – Fred Astaire or Darcey Bussell – or a sportsperson such as a gymnast, rugby player or skateboarder. I love to watch the *Strictly* professionals that I work with – they're a major inspiration for me. Make time to watch someone who carries joy in the way they move and imagine what that must feel like. Remember that imagined feeling when you turn on some music and start your routine for the day – get into the rhythm of the moves and concentrate on how your body is moving in different ways.

Ready, Steady, Cook!

How do you feel about cooking? Is it something that gives you joy or fills you with dread? Or is it great when you have the time and the energy but something that often isn't top of your list? Today, I want you to plan to cook one meal from scratch this week. Or one more meal than usual.

It doesn't have to be elaborate or expensive – pick something simple that you can create with all natural ingredients that will nourish your body. For example, ditch the packet sauce that you put in your stir-fry for something homemade. Find an appetizing one-pot meal or slow cooker/crock-pot recipe that can cook while you're getting on with something else. Plan ahead so that you can look forward to a meal that will make you happy (and perhaps leave some leftovers for lunch the next day).

Journaling

As I talked about earlier (see page 44), journaling is another way to look at our intentions and our feelings around the subject of movement. It can help us identify what is helping and hindering us on our journey toward finding the joy in moving our bodies.

Try the prompts given for each week, or take some time each day to think about movement and health and what they mean to you, and how you could build a stronger relationship with your body.

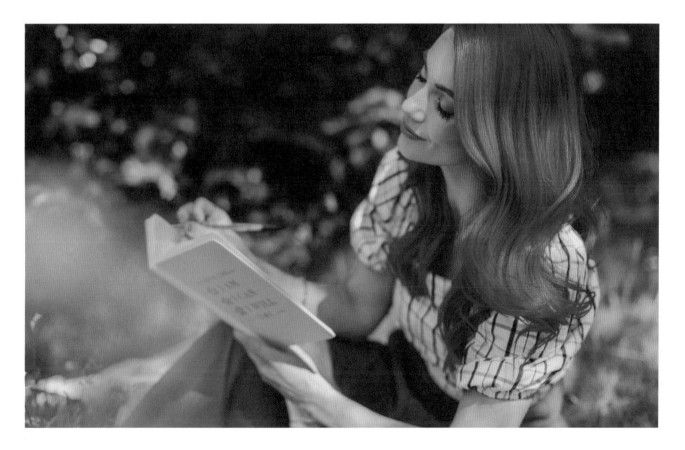

**JOURNALLING
PROMPT**

First and foremost, why did I decide to start this journey? What encouraged me? How do I want to feel at the end of the three weeks?

DAY 3

Earthing Energy Booster

I love the concept of the Earth giving us energy. Try sitting, standing or lying in different poses where your bare skin is in contact with the Earth. Feel the energy coming up from the floor and through your body, giving you an extra boost of strength.

Warm-up: Cat-Cow x 8

- Donkey Kicks with Push-up Variation x 8
- Downward Dog for 3–5 breaths
- High Lunge with Cactus Arms on right with Low Lunge Variation x 8
- Downward Dog for 3–5 breaths
- High Lunge with Cactus Arms on left with Low Lunge Variation x 8
- Downward Dog for 3–5 breaths
- Cat-Cow x 4

Cool down: Lying Spine Twist for 5 breaths, or however long feels good

Getting Started

Everyone knows that the hardest part of anything is getting started. What are your barriers? What might be holding you back?

This plan is about doing it for yourself – all for you and nobody else. Sometimes taking that time just for you can prompt so many more things to start happening in your life because you are putting time and effort into yourself.

Make sure you're planning the best time to fit the routine into your day. How is it going so far? Can you find ways to make exercise even easier for tomorrow – having exercise clothing to hand or making sure that your morning routine allows you enough time for yourself? Start tracking your steps on your cellphone now so you can be more aware of how much you are moving each day.

Feel Your Food

This plan is not about dieting or restricting yourself. I want you to think about what you're eating and how you're feeling. Keep an eye on what foods make you feel a certain way. Say you have a massive bowl of pasta – how do you feel afterwards? Energetic or sluggish? It's important to be aware of how the foods you're eating are impacting on your body – positively or negatively. Are you getting protein, carbs and plenty of fruit and veggies onto your plate? Do you sit down for three meals a day or grab bites on the move? Do you feel satisfied after a good meal, and do you feel hungry before a meal? Practise eating at regular times and see if it changes how you feel and what foods you crave.

Eight Hours!

Sleep is such a crucial aspect to improve your movement and overall health. A lack of sleep affects everything – from the hormones that influence our food cravings, to our energy levels and desire to do our daily five minutes of yoga, as well as our overall mindset and mood. Most adults need between seven and ten hours of sleep each night, but many of us have compromised sleep habits. Do yourself a favour and find the time for sufficient sleep – set up a sleep routine to gain the full health benefits and take note of the positive effects it has on your life.

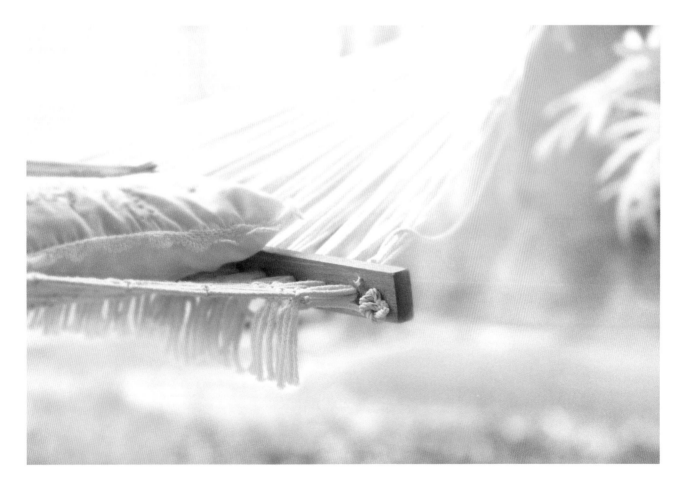

DAY 4

Yoga for Stress Relief

We're all exposed to stress and pressure every day and we hold so much tension in our bodies and minds. This routine works on both our muscles and our minds by encouraging our bodies to relax, helping us to feel calmer and more in control. Taking a moment to do something for your wellbeing is important, so this is one of my favourite routines.

Warm-up: Cat–Cow x 8

- Dead Bug with Knee to Elbow Variation x 8
- Lying Spine Twist on right for 3–5 breaths
- Knees to Chest for 3–5 breaths
- Lying Spine Twist on left for 3–5 breaths
- Tabletop Arms and Legs x 4 on each side
- Child's Pose for 1 breath
- Downward Dog for 3–5 breaths
- Right One-legged Dog into
- High Lunge with Cactus Arms, right leg forward for 3 breaths
- Triangle Pose on the right for 1 breath
- Standing Forward Fold for 1 breath
- Mountain Pose for 1 breath
- Tree Pose on the right for 1 breath
- Downward Dog for 1 breath
- Go again from the One-legged Dog, repeating all on the left leg

Cool down: Happy Baby for 8–10 breaths, or however long feels good

Joyful Movement

Think about your favourite sports and activities from when you were a child. Trampolining? Skipping? Skateboarding? Football? Tag?

What did you play in the school playground? Or when you met up with friends? As adults, we forget about the active fun that came naturally to us as children. Think about how to bring that enjoyment back into your life. Get a rebounder if not a trampoline. Join an adult sports or gymnastics club. Visit a climbing wall or an indoor ski centre. Think about and research some options to try out new hobbies and ways to play!

Drink More Water

We all know that we should drink more water, and yet it's something that takes effort. Make a plan to increase the water you drink every day. Perhaps chill a jug of water so that you always have cold water available if you don't work near a watercooler. Perhaps you could decide to drink a glass of water for every hot drink you have this week. Look for easy ways to bring water into your day without having to think about it.

Rest Up

Almost as important as healthy sleep habits is finding time in your day and week for rest. Is this something you consider or prioritize?

The more balance and space you can bring into your life, the easier it will be to make the necessary decisions to protect your own time and energy. Ensure that your day isn't all about work and others – some of it needs to be self-centred. Use your diary to plan half an hour before or after work, lunch or dinner for a walk in nature, or 30 minutes resting with a book or an extra ten minutes of yoga to relax and wind down.

"We all know that we should drink more water, and yet it's something that takes effort. Make a plan to increase the water you drink every day."

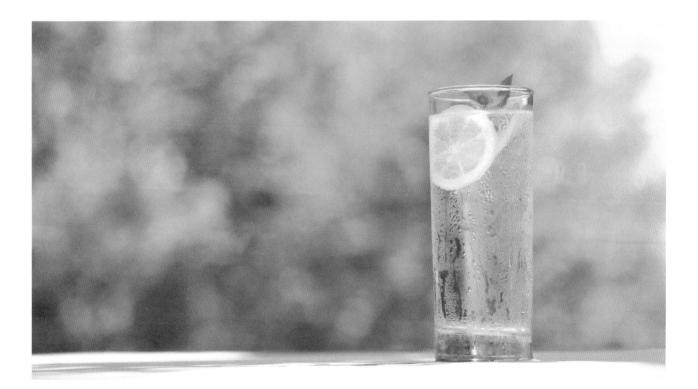

DAY 5

Sculpt and Tone Pilates

Pilates is so good for working on the alignment of your body – one of the reasons I love it. Here you really focus on lengthening the muscles and your body's positioning. It will sculpt and tone the muscles you didn't realize were working, and also help you to remember how your body should feel when it's properly aligned – useful when you're tempted to slouch at your desk or slump on the sofa.

Warm-up: Dead Bug with Knee to Elbow Variation x 8 on each side

- Bridge Pose with Dips Variation x 8
- Reverse Bridge with Leg Lift x 4 on each side
- Lying Leg Scissor Kicks x 8
- Oblique Curls x 8
- Corkscrew x 2
- Mountain Climbers x 10

Cool down: Lizard Lunge with Arm Variation x 2 on each side

Little and Often

Today I want you to actively think about the power of the incidental exercise you take during the day that gets your body moving, twisting and turning. I want you to focus on, appreciate and "bank" the exercise you're doing and enjoy it.

Be aware of the opportunities to move every day and look for those little extras you can do – taking the option to walk to the train station, walking the dog, weeding a garden border or mopping the floor vigorously. Consider these little things you do to keep your body moving without even being particularly conscious of it – activities you might try to avoid, or not exactly look forward to, but only take five minutes and you've moved your body. Think about how your body is moving and focus on the muscles that are stretching and flexing as you maximize this exercise.

New Tastes

Why not pick up a new natural food item today at the store? Try a different fruit or vegetable and source a recipe for it – or perhaps try a spice or herb you haven't cooked with before. It's easy to stick to what we know, but there are wonderful flavours out there that need to be tried. This isn't about being an adventurous eater or trying something exotic – just about being open to new ideas. Whether it's sweet potato or ginger, grapefruit or pinto beans – look on the shelf next to your usual favourites and get experimenting with something new.

Up with the Lark

Sleep is important but the morning hours bring precious opportunities to look after your body. Try waking up reasonably early and getting outside first thing in the morning, absorbing the natural light as well as some fresh air. Increased time in natural light ensures you max out on Vitamin D (essential for so many of our bodily systems), improves mood and helps regulate the body's circadian rhythms to enhance our quality of sleep. Plus the benefits of natural light on our ability to focus and be productive have been proven – studies have shown that workers sitting next to a window are more productive than those working away from natural light. Also avoiding tech for the first and last hours of the day has a positive influence on your sleep quality (and is a great way to ringfence your time). I feel so much better for my morning light boost while I walk around the garden before breakfast every day.

Stop using your phone an hour or two before bed so you're able to get to sleep 15 minutes earlier. That way you'll be able to wake up a little earlier to do your exercise, plus you'll get more deep sleep and be able to function better during the day.

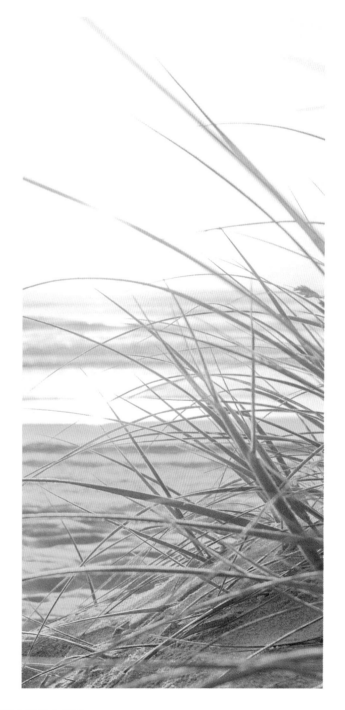

DAY 6

Burner Cardio

Cardio exercise is great for your cardiovascular system. You don't need to do cardio every day, but it's great to get your heart rate up two or three times a week. I do my cardio workouts for my heart, but it also gives me a really good feeling afterwards and helps me mentally. A boost of endorphins is great if I'm in a low mood. I'll tend to go for something cardio-based on those days and there's such satisfaction in having pushed yourself.

Warm-up: Chair Pose with Calf Raise Variation x 4

- First to Second Position Squat Jumps x 20
- Curtsy Squats x 10 on each side
- Dead Bug with Knee to Elbow Variation x 15
- Mountain Climbers for 30 seconds
- Double Straight Leg Stretch x 10
- Repeat the routine as needed

Cool down: Hip Rolls x 10

Get out in Nature

Getting outside for some exercise is fantastic in so many ways. Whether you're walking, gardening, running, swimming or cycling, the fresh air is good for mind and body.

Adding something simple like a ten-minute walk into your lunch-hour is an easy way to start increasing your daily activity levels. Make plans for a couple of outdoor walks or activities over the next few days.

What's in my Food?

Start thinking more about what you're eating and what it contains. Many packaged foods that we grab to eat on the move are packed full of preservatives, salt, sugars, artificial flavourings and thickeners, while also being lower in fibre, protein and vitamins and minerals than the real deal. Low-fat foods are often lower in fat but compensate with salt and sugar instead. Labels on foods help you to think about the food choices you make – look at the number of strange ingredients that often appear on labels and try to eat more foods in their whole form – foods that have no labels. Educate yourself about good food choices and fill your plate with foods to nourish your body. A plain jacket potato is a healthy and filling carbohydrate meal, but a pile of chips that weighs the same is full of saturated fats, while crisps are heavily salted. Plain oatmeal with berries and natural peanut butter contains no sugar, but some breakfast cereals contain up to five spoonfuls in one serving. There is twice as much sugar in a glass of orange juice as in an orange itself.

Colour my Life

Be colourful today – put on a different colour that you don't normally wear and enjoy the way it makes you feel. Eat more colour too. It's scientifically proven that eating a wider selection of colours of fruits and vegetables increases the variety of super-soothing phytonutrients that we receive – the natural chemicals found in plants that protect them and us from chronic disease and environmental threat. There are five "colour types": red (good for heart health), green (helps detoxify), purple (supports the nervous system), yellow (for improved mood) and orange (to beat inflammation). Focus on bringing colour into your day.

> "Be colourful today – put on a different colour that you don't normally wear and enjoy the way it makes you feel."

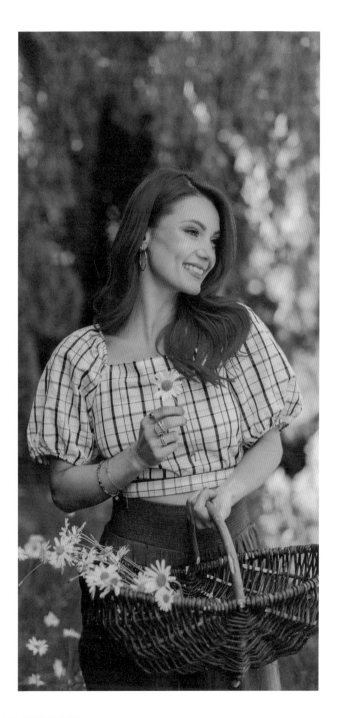

DAY 7

Awakening Flow

A morning flow is good for body and mind. How you start the day can set up your mood and determine how the rest of your day goes. So if you can do something really positive in the morning, and for yourself, you'll be in a stronger position to feel more alive and energized all day, and to help others.

Warm-up: Knees to Chest with Standing Variation for 3 breaths on each side

- Mountain Pose for 1 breath
- Standing Forward Fold for 1 breath
- Halfway Lift for 3–5 breaths
- Tabletop Arms and Legs x 4 on each side
- Downward Dog for 3–5 breaths
- One-legged Dog on right for 3–5 breaths
- Warrior 1 on right for 3–5 breaths
- Warrior 2 on right for 3–5 breaths
- Forearm Plank to Straight Arm Plank x 8
- Downward Dog for 3–5 breaths
- Repeat routine on the left

Cool down: Lying Knees to Chest for 8–10 breaths, or however long feels good

Listen to Your Body

At the end of Week 1, what days were easy/hard? Which of the routines did you enjoy the most? Which lifestyle ideas clicked? Be proud of yourself for completing your first week.

For Week 2 maybe you could set your alarm ten minutes earlier to fit in some extra stretches or movement in the morning. Or can you find time in your lunch break to do a few minutes of meditation? Look for opportunities to make time for yourself – to rest or to move your body.

One More on the Plate

Today, add one extra vegetable to your main meal, or eat an extra portion of fruit. Remember the concept of "crowding out" (see page 23) and make sure to fill your plate with vegetables and fruit.

Various studies have shown that a diet including ten vegetable and fruit portions a day cuts your risk of a range of chronic illnesses, including all kinds of cancer, by up to one third. Ten portions is a lot to achieve, but just adding one more is a step toward a healthier lifestyle.

Celebrate the Day

Look after and be grateful for your body today. Celebrate the end of Week 1 and treat yourself with a massage or perhaps try out body brushing (exfoliating and massaging your skin with a special firm-bristled brush) at home. Look for nourishing rituals that make you feel good.

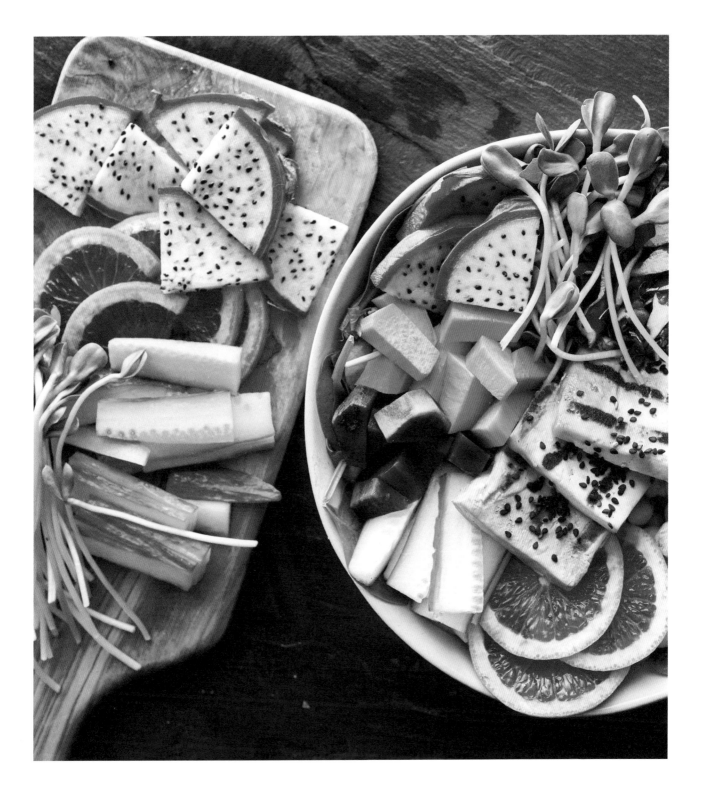

Week 2

Routine

MANTRA

I am strong, I believe in myself.

DAY 8

Arms and Abs

This is a super-important toning routine. A strong core is essential for healthy body movement. If your core is strong, then you're more effective when using your arms and legs and during all forms of exercise. Everything is aligned when your core is working properly – a strong core leads to a strong back and good posture.

Warm-up: First to Second Position Squat Jumps with arms out for 30–60 seconds

- Downward Dog into
- Plank with Straight Arm Variation into
- Chaturanga (Low Plank) into
- Upward Dog into
- Plank with Straight Arm Variation
- Repeat the above 5 exercises as a flow combination x 8
- Dead Bug x 8
- Oblique Curls x 8
- Dead Bug with Knee to Elbow Variation x 8
- Plank for 30–60 seconds
- Repeat entire routine 2–4 times

Cool down: Lying Spine Twist for 8–10 breaths on each side, or however long feels good

Getting into a Routine

What is your exercise routine looking like so far? Think about ways to improve and embed your movement habits in Week 2.

As well as the routines, choose one move, exercise or pose for the week to practise every day, with a reps or time target. Hip opening ones are really good for this, as you can improve on them and soon feel the difference – like in Happy Baby (page 124) when you can pull your knees further down. Or try perfecting your Standing Forward Fold (page 127) – start with knees bent and see how they become straighter with practise.

Get Prepping

Start Week 2 by making a list of ideas for healthy meals and snacks you can prep for the week ahead. Having something good for you ready to grab is the easiest way to ensure that you pack your diet with great choices – and save yourself time and money as well.

I might make a veggie chilli or stew – something that tastes better the day after you've made it, or perhaps some homemade pesto that keeps in the fridge for a few days. Energy balls – with oats and dried fruits – are always in my fridge too. Make good use of your fridge and freezer to fill your diet with colourful options.

Wheel of Life

Now is a good time to draw up your own Wheel of Life if you haven't already (see page 45). Select the areas of your life that are important to you and chart out the week ahead. What time do you have to spend with family or friends? What about creative projects or hobbies? Ensure that sleep and rest are properly accounted for too. If you don't have time for all of these, look at why not – what is filling up time that should be used for non-work/play/rest/sleep? You could journal around what is taking up more or less time than you expected and why this might be.

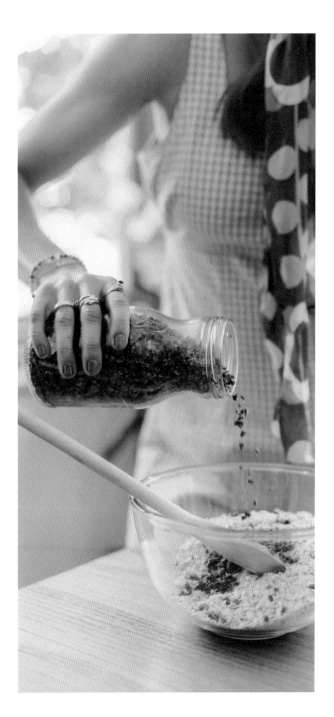

**JOURNALING
PROMPT**

**What am I enjoying so far
with the plan? How do the
changes make me feel?**

DAY 9

Inspired Jive

Jive was one of my favourite dances growing up purely because of the energy levels. It's always the last dance that you do in a competition so you can put all of your energy into it and have the best time doing it. People find this dance one of the most physically exhausting because it's fast and your feet are constantly moving – it's like you're running up a hill for 1 minute 30 when we do it on *Strictly*!

Warm-up: Jump Back With Clap x 8

- Forward and Side Kicks x 8 each side
- Chassé x 4 each side
- Shuffle Ball Heel x 2 each side
- Jump Back with Clap x 8

Cool down: Standing Forward Fold with Ragdoll for 8–10 breaths, or however long feels good

Manifesting

Manifestation is a big thing for me. It's all about defining what you really want and how you're going to get there. Think about your exercise – what is it that you want to achieve? Define that clear goal – one thing – and consider how you can make that happen, or what steps can you take toward your goal? It is possible if you put your mind to it. Accountability is also key. Why not start by writing down your goal and the steps you need to take to achieve it? You can put it somewhere you'll see it every day to remind yourself.

Intuitive Eating

Intuitive eating is about listening to your body and what it tells you it wants. For the next two to three days, try to eat with your body, without limiting yourself, and remembering that you don't have to eat at certain times or eat certain amounts. Obviously if you feel hungry it's a sign that your body needs some nutritious food – and the key word here is nutritious. Give your body good quality food and you will see a difference in your eating habits. Also, enjoy your eating. Sit at the table and eat at leisure. Light a candle or put some music on. Turn off your phone and concentrate on eating with all your senses. Eat with other people where possible.

Being Present

Mindfulness supports us to work at tuning out the busyness of our brains to focus on the here and now. Experiment with simple hacks like putting your phone on mute and leaving it to one side for a couple of hours at a time, eating slowly and savouring every bite, or go for a walk in nature without any other distractions and take in the sights, sounds and smells of the natural world. Learning to enjoy the moment takes constant practice but the benefits are fantastic for our mental health and happiness.

"...go for a walk in nature without any other distractions and take in the sights, sounds and smells of the natural world."

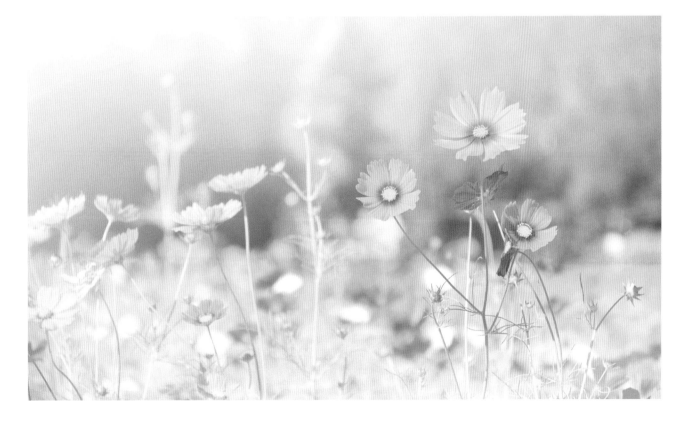

DAY 10

Stretch Yoga

I can't over-emphasize how important stretching is for our bodies, especially for me as a dancer. Stretching supports your body around working out and improves your range of movement. I like to stretch before and after workouts as sometimes a workout can put your body under pressure, so calming the body down before and after is essential. This is a lovely stretch for the morning after we've hopefully been asleep for eight hours.

Warm-up: Puppy Pose for 3–5 breaths

- Downward Dog for 3–5 breaths
- One-legged Dog on right for 3–5 breaths
- Lizard Stretch on right for 3–5 breaths
- Plié Squat for 3–5 breaths
- Side Lunges on right x 4
- Standing Forward Fold x 2
- Chair Pose with Calf Raise Variation on the right x 4
- Repeat the routine on the left

Cool down: Happy Baby for 8–10 breaths, or however long feels good

Incidental Exercise #2

Remember the Blue Zone areas we discussed earlier (see page 13).

These people with their prime health have probably never been to a gym in their life. Their "gym workout" is walking to get their fresh vegetables, picking them and cooking them simply at home. Their leisure time is filled with family and friends, and all of that comes together to create a healthy life. Rather than finding time to put in an hour at the gym twice this week, listen to your body. If you have more energy, then of course you could do some more stretches and exercise. If you're tired, then listen to what your body needs. Look for ways to be more active while living a life true to your own priorities.

Green Day

Go veggie or vegan for the day, if you're not already. Trialing a different eating style or choice is a great way to bring new cooking methods and ingredients into your daily life. It will also help you see what works for your body, or not. Being in tune with your body is key to understanding what foods fuel you and which ones don't make you feel as good. For example, I've discovered that tomatoes give me stomach pains and make me feel sluggish so I avoid them although they're great for other people.

Be Mindful

Today is a good day to support your soothing yoga practice with five minutes of meditation. Remember that it takes a while to get into the rhythm of meditation, so why not start with a simple seated sound meditation? Choose a quiet place and time of day and select a sound to listen to – perhaps waves or rainfall. Otherwise, just listen to the sounds around you. Close your eyes and focus, trying to keep your mind on the sound. If you find your mind wandering, just calmly bring it back to your body and the sound. Set a timer for five minutes if necessary.

Try out a few meditation apps if you find that easier. The best meditation is always the sort that you will find time to do regularly.

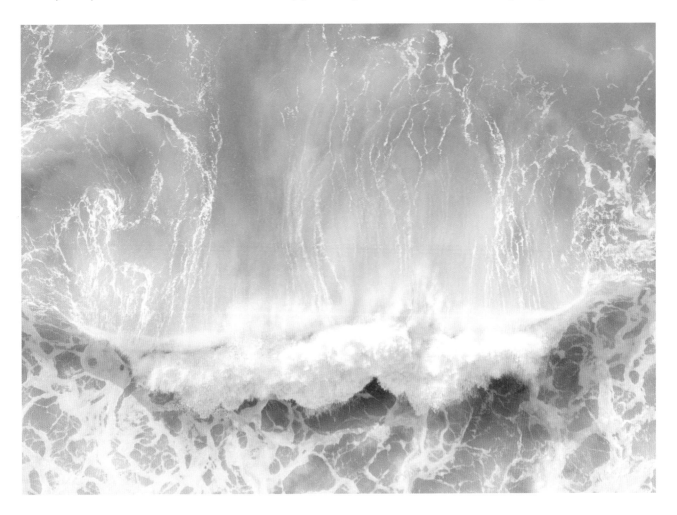

DAY 11

Legs and Core Supersets

This is a more challenging and high-intensity routine. Leg movements are something I struggle with, and I'm told that adding strength into my legs means that my lower back and glutes work better. So here your core is doing a lot of the work but you're also working on the muscles in and around your legs.

Warm-up: slow Plié Squats x 10

Superset 1:
- Chair Pose with double Calf Raise Variation x 8
- Tabletop Arms and Legs x 8 on each side

Superset 2:
- Lying Leg Circles x 8 on each side
- Lying Leg Scissor Kicks x 8

Superset 3:
- Plié Squats x 8
- Lizard Lunge to Plank x 4 on each side, holding each lunge for 1 breath

Superset 4:
- Donkey Kicks x 8 on each side
- Lying Leg Scissor Kicks x 8

Repeat all of the sets 2–3 times

Cool down: Half Pigeon for 8–10 breaths on each side, or however long feels good

Posture

Today, think about your posture – we all sit a lot of the time, and often in a non-posture-friendly way. Be aware of your body's alignment: how are you sitting when you're on the train or at your desk?

Posture is important in Pilates and yoga – take what you can from these disciplines and try to remember to engage your core and keep your spine upright and aligned when you're sitting down. It'll benefit your physical body, and studies have shown surprising benefits of good posture on your mental health too. Standing or sitting tall can make us feel more positive and powerful, and affects our hormone levels.

Also look for ways to bring in simple exercises when you're inactive. For example, when you're sitting down regularly, lift one leg then the other using your core. Or try a Mountain Pose or Forward Fold when you're standing next to the kettle.

Dust off Your Herbs and Spices

Add extra flavour to your homecooked food with a superfood addition. There are a host of spices and herbs that improve flavour and are great for you.

Turmeric has numerous scientifically-proven benefits – it's beneficial for heart health and may help with depression and arthritis along with having anti-inflammatory properties. I add it to scrambled eggs in the morning or a homemade latte. Cacao powder tastes like dark chocolate and is packed with flavonoids, which work on your blood pressure and blood health. It's said to have three times the level of antioxidants of green tea, along with high levels of magnesium and sulphur – pop it in a smoothie or spread it on toast. Cardamom, nutmeg, ginger and cinnamon are also supercharged additions to oatmeal, smoothies or sprinkled on fruit to add natural sweetness.

Similarly, look for ways to cook with your favourite herbs or use them as garnishes. They're easy to grow in the garden or on the windowsill.

Find the Beat

You've been enjoying some different music so far while trialing the routines. How do the different styles make you feel while you move? Do they energize you and make your movement time more fun? Find some pumping anthems that make you push through an energetic routine, or a calming rhythmic instrumental for a soothing yoga flow. Spend some time today creating a playlist of dynamic or soothing tunes to dance, exercise or walk to over the coming days, and commit to regularly changing it up.

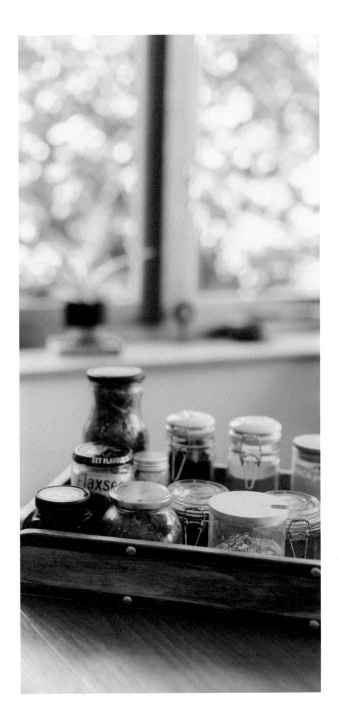

DAY 12

Dancer's Contemporary Flow

In this routine, try to move through all the positions without stopping. In a normal yoga flow you can be a little stiffer in your movements, but in this one my aim is to let nothing have a "button" on the end – every movement should just flow into the next. Think of it like yoga but with a dance element added.

Warm-up: Standing Forward Fold x 4

- Ragdoll with Swing into
- Standing Leg Lifts x 8 each side
- High Lunge with right leg forward for 3–5 breaths
- High Lunge with left leg forward for 3–5 breaths
- Standing Leg Lifts x 8 each side
- Standing Forward Fold into
- Halfway Lift into
- Half Splits x 4 each side
- Repeat the routine

Cool down: Lying Spine Twist for 10 breaths, or however long feels good

Kitchen Disco

Today, just choose a brilliant song that puts a big smile on your face and dance round the kitchen as if no one is watching. Have a crazy moment and let go. Relish the moment and how it makes you feel. Love the movement!

Breakfast like a King

Breakfast is probably my favourite meal and such a great way to start the day, but it's the meal when people often just have the same thing every day.

Why not change it up a little? We don't eat the same thing for lunch or dinner every day so play with some different options for breakfast – cook eggs in different ways and add extras like spinach or mushrooms. Try smoothies or yogurt with fruits and toppings. Focus on protein, fruit and veg and healthy fats for a meal that keeps you satisfied all morning and helps you avoid unhealthy snacking.

Say "No" More

Look at your diary for the coming weeks and do some decluttering. Saying "no" is so important – stop thinking of "shoulds" and concentrate on nourishing your priorities in life. Finding a way to gracefully say "Thanks but no thanks" at the outset is respectful of both parties. Use the line "That sounds great, but my diary is jammed at the moment. I'll let you know tomorrow" to give you the space to consider whether you can commit or not.

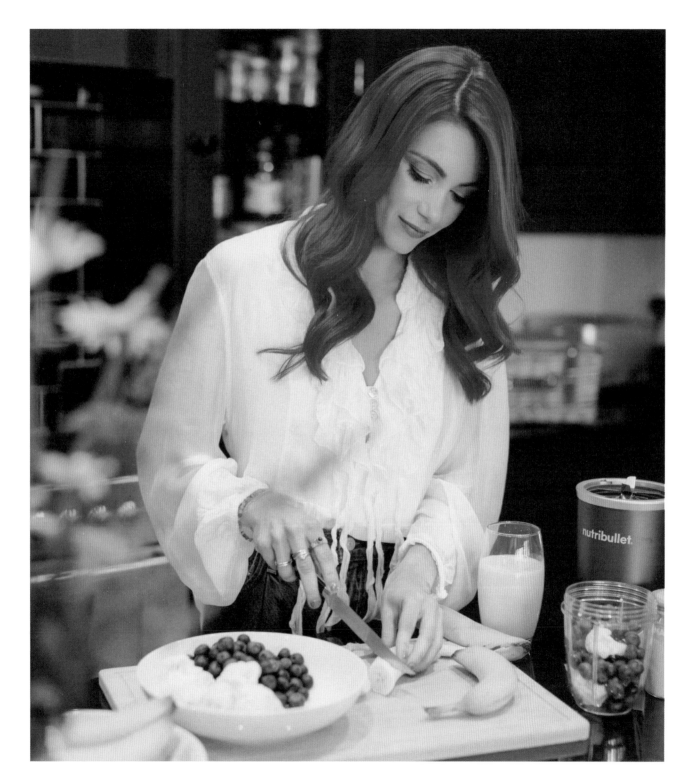

DAY 13

Hip Opener

If we're sitting a lot all day, our hips aren't really doing that much and can get stuck in a stagnant position. I have problems with my hips, so hip openers are essential for me to keep my hips healthy and moving effectively for my dancing. It's like when you oil a bike chain – doing a nice hip opener flow helps keep your hips and surrounding muscles healthy.

Warm-up: Happy Baby for 8–10 breaths

- Downward Dog with Twist Variation x 4 each side
- Lizard Lunge with Arm Stretch Variation (right arm to ceiling) for 3–5 breaths
- Straight Arm Plank for 1 breath
- Lizard Lunge with Arm Stretch Variation (left arm to ceiling) for 3–5 breaths
- Lying Knees to Chest (each leg, then both legs together) for 3–5 breaths
- Lying Spine Twist for 3–5 breaths
- Repeat the routine if you can

Cool down: Half Pigeon for 8–10 breaths on each side, or however long feels good

Weight-Bearing Exercise

Weight-bearing exercise – especially simple moves using your own body weight – are crucial for healthy bones, particularly as you get older. Prioritize easy ways to bring more weight-bearing exercise into your daily life – it can be as simple as climbing stairs and walking. You could also use everyday fitness equipment such as a skipping rope (ten minutes a day) or an exercise band or weights (such as milk cartons, a full water bottle or I did some lifting with my small niece recently!). Have fun and try out different ideas out while the kettle boils.

Wholefoods

The best foods for us are items that are eaten in their original form – one-ingredient food items. They're the staple of every healthy eating plan. What actually is a wholefood? Fruit and veg, pulses, meat and fish, nuts and seeds, eggs, grains, herbs and spices haven't been modified, so they're wholefoods. Learn how to cook dishes based around these items. It doesn't have to be fancy food using 25 ingredients – master some simple dishes with your favourite foods. Top tip – frozen veg is a fantastic staple to have in for when you've not had time to get fresh veg from the shops.

Get Creative

Look at how and when you indulge creativity in your life and what opportunities you have to get your brain working in a different way. From painting to crossword puzzles, gardening to making cards, ensure that your Wheel of Life (see page 45) includes some time to indulge in your hobbies. If you need to find new creative avenues, think back to your childhood. What did you enjoy doing in your spare time – colouring, crafting, collecting things or playing an instrument? Play with some ideas to find out what makes you happy.

"Look at how and when you indulge creativity in your life and what opportunities you have to get your brain working in a different way."

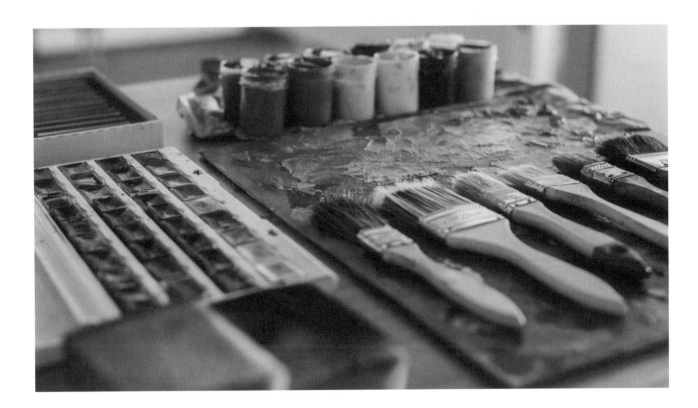

DAY 14

Rest Day Restorative Yoga

Rest is so important for your mental and physical health, so it's essential to dedicate a day, or at least part of a day, to resting your mind and body. Try to fit in a complete rest day at least once a month. We don't give downtime enough attention – we always focus on doing, doing, doing. Even just sitting in front of the TV means that your mind is still active and watching the programme (and you're probably checking your social media at the same time too), so with this routine really enjoy the yoga and try to take your mind to a resting place.

Begin lying down, then hold each pose for 6–8 solid breaths.

Warm-up: Puppy Pose for 8–10 breaths

- Child's Pose with Raised Arm Variation x 2 on each side
- Half Pigeon on each side
- Warrior 1 on each side
- Warrior 2 on each side
- Tree Pose on each side
- Repeat the routine

Cool down: Lying Spine Twist on each side for 8–10 breaths, or however long feels good

New Moves

At two weeks in, you have tried a wide range of the exercise routines now. I hope you're feeling and seeing a difference in your body. Think about what your favourite workout has been so far, and if that is something you might add into your everyday routine – consider what you enjoyed, as that's what you're more likely to do again.

New Tastes

You've tried new patterns of eating and trialed different foods this week. What have you learned about enjoying your food? What has been the most effective and simple tip for eating better? Look at what has worked for you – whether it's trying new foods, prepping dishes ahead of time or changing elements of your diet.

Good Habits

At the end of Week 2, I hope that your diary is starting to look different than at the beginning of the plan. Notice what you are adding and taking away from the days. What parts of your day have made you feel lightest and at your best this past week? How is meditation and creativity fitting into your life? What habits are you going to build on for the future?

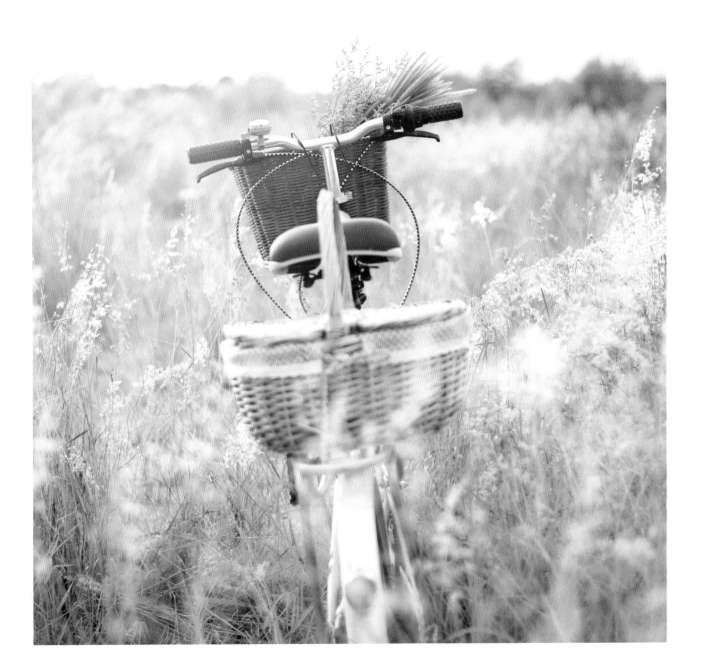

Week 3

Set your Goals

MANTRA

I'm doing this for me.
Our intentions create
our reality.

DAY 15

Power Routine

This intensive routine picks up the pace. You're aiming for full power, but it's key to make sure to keep your alignment and technique as it should be. I'd rather you did fewer reps if it means keeping your form.

Warm-up: 4 x "walk outs". Stretch into an Upward Dog then walk your hands back toward your feet and roll up to standing.

Each move takes one minute – spend 45 seconds on the move and take 15 seconds rest.

- Plié Squats – hold your arms overhead
- Donkey Kicks with Push-Up Variation (alternate between each side)
- Dead Bug with Knee to Elbow Variation
- High Lunge with right leg forward up to standing, then to Warrior 3, then back to standing. Repeat on the left side.
- Mountain Climbers
- Repeat the routine 2–3 times

Cool down: Hip Rolls for 30–60 seconds

Exercise Snacking

I love the idea of snatching snippets of time for exercise when you can't commit to large chunks of time.

If you don't have a full hour in your day, then break it up and try for little and often. Do five minutes in the morning and ten minutes at lunchtime. Everyone can manage a five-minute workout – there is no excuse not to do that. And it's better to put all your effort into five minutes of exercise, and get that great feeling afterwards, than waiting until you have an hour free and just coasting through it as you're not really in the mood.

New Cuisine

Choose a cuisine from another country to explore today – selecting a couple of ingredients or a dish to make that you've not tried before. This should feel an attractive challenge after the new tastes you've been trialing. Remember that this is about having fun with food and not about making life difficult.

Into the Routine

Whether it's exercise first thing or celebrating your sleep time, why not trial a morning and/or evening routine that brings together your mantra and journaling plus some screen-free time to top and tail your day? Creating space at the beginning and end of the day helps you to focus your intention and mindset without being dragged into other people's needs, and it helps you make YOU the focus of your time.

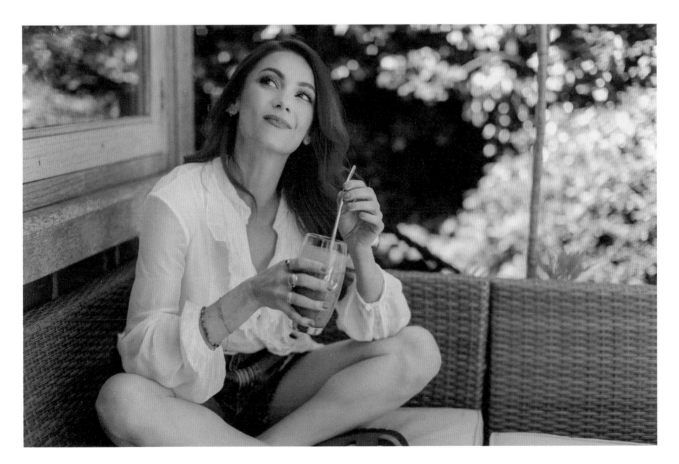

DAY 16

Tap

I started tap dance later than ballroom, but I love the way you create the rhythm with your body. Once I got into tap, I found I was tapping away and didn't realize until later that my legs were burning, as you use your leg muscles so much. It's such a great leg strengthener but also just so much fun.

Warm-up: slow Plié Squats x 10

- Ball Heel right and Ball Heel left x 8 alternating
- Shuffle Tap right and Shuffle Tap left x 8 alternating
- Shuffle Ball Heel right and Shuffle Ball Heel left x 8 alternating
- Cross Shuffle Ball Heel right and Cross Shuffle Ball Heel left x 8 alternating
- Repeat the routine 2–4 times

Cool down: Pigeon Pose for 8–10 breaths on each side, or however long feels good

Find an Exercise Buddy

Try to find an exercise partner or just call up a friend to come and walk with you. Again – how many times can I say the word? – look for the JOY in exercising. It's true, you may not rack up quite the same amount of heart-pumping exercise with someone else as you would by yourself, but the point is that you'll have a good time. You definitely won't decide at the last minute that you can't do it. And you'll do it again. It's a no-brainer.

Eat Sustainably

Can you come up with three new ways of eating sustainably?

Are you in a position to start your own veg patch or make your own oat milk or create something from scratch that you would normally buy? Why not visit a fruit farm to pick your own, pickle some veg for a healthy kimchi or learn about preserving so that you can reduce leftovers and eat more economically? There is a real satisfaction in growing vegetables or fruit and harvesting your own homegrown produce – helping the planet and eating better at the same time.

Screen-Free Day

Quite simply, put down your phone and be more present. If it's not possible to sign off from the digital world for the day, then schedule a day when it is possible. In the meantime, try to build a couple of two-hour slots into your day when you're screen-free but contactable in an emergency. Use your out-of-office to step away from ongoing notifications if it helps.

Look at your relationship with your tech to see what you can do to try to be more present in your life every day.

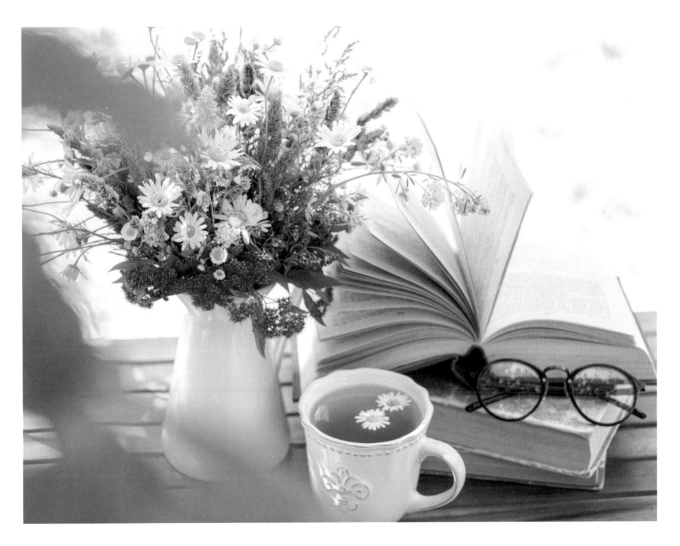

DAY 17

Heart Opener Yoga

This is another great stress reliever routine. When we're working all day, we may be crunching up our bodies or slouching without realizing and it's great to reverse that feeling. You'll be surprised at how energizing this kind of movement can be; getting blood to the centre of the chest while being a lovely stretch for your heart space. This is a flow routine, so hold each pose for 3-5 breaths.

Warm-up: Happy Baby for 8-10 breaths

- Tabletop Arms and Legs x 4 on each side alternating
- Downward Dog into
- Warrior 2 into
- Triangle Pose into
- Mountain Pose into
- Standing Forward Fold into
- Straight Arm Plank into
- Chaturanga (Low Plank) into
- Upward Dog into
- Downward Dog into
- Wild Thing on right leg into
- Downward Dog into
- Low Lunge with Cactus Arms on right into
- Downward Dog
- Repeat the routine on the left side

Cool down: Lying Spine Twist for 8-10 breaths, or however long feels good

Walk More

Count how many steps you've done over the past week or so – and make a plan to take them up a level. Noting your step count with your phone or tracker is a great way to become more aware of how much you're moving, and whether your lifestyle is active or you are actually sitting down a lot of the time. Ask yourself: do I need to add something to my day to get my body moving more? Can I add five minutes at the beginning or end of the day? Can I walk to the station three times a week? Consistency is key – slow and steady wins the race.

Add Another Vegetable or Fruit to Your Plate

Take your veg and fruit intake up a notch again by adding one more extra portion to your day – maybe another veg snack option, a smoothie for breakfast or lunch, a small salad with a meal or bulk out a curry with another veg. It's easy and becomes a habit if you look at meals and snacks as opportunities for ways to crowd out your plate with goodness.

Get Grateful

The wonderful thing about practicing gratitude is how it helps you to notice the small, simple things that lift your days. It becomes easier to put a positive spin on situations and view them as opportunities. Not everything is going to go your way – that is life – but if you can be grateful for all that you have, then you will find your days feel better and you're more positive about your life in general. Try a gratitude diary or just spend 30 seconds thinking of three positive aspects to your day as you climb into bed. Scientists have shown that those who find time for a regular gratitude practice sleep better, exercise more and are happier than those who don't. It's a must.

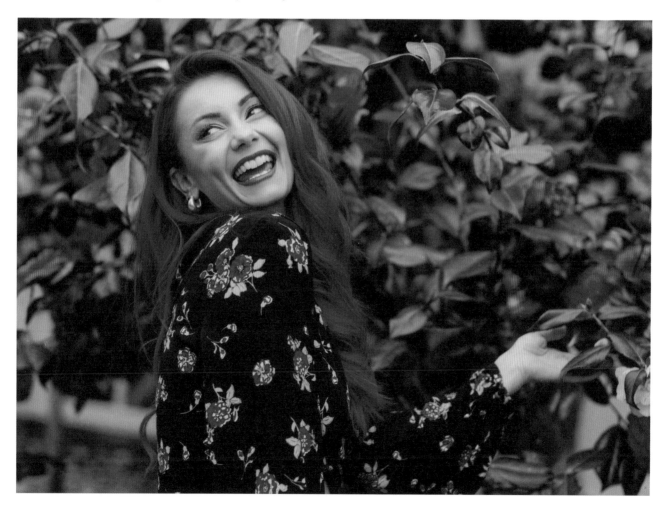

DAY 18

Pilates Ballet Fit

Pilates and ballet go hand in hand – a lot of what you learn in ballet crosses over with Pilates, from the similar ways of standing to the importance of alignment. Many ballerinas do Pilates work for strength, and vice versa. I found that adding Pilates and ballet to my routine really helps my Latin and ballroom. It's amazing how you can do the smallest and simplest moves and really feel the effects the next day.

Warm-up: Child's Pose for 8–10 breaths

- Arm Circles x 16 in each direction
- Arms Serving Food x 16
- Arms Up and Down x 16
- Arms Criss Cross x 16
- Calf Raises x 8 on each leg
- First to Second Position Squat Jumps x 8 on each leg
- Standing Leg Lifts x 8 in each direction on each leg
- Lying Leg Scissor Kicks x 16
- Double Straight Leg Stretch
- Repeat the routine 2–4 times

Cool down: Knee to Chest for 30–60 seconds each side, or however long feels good

New Moves

Dance, yoga and Pilates tick lots of boxes in terms of health benefits plus the ease at which they can be picked up at home. But now I want you to think about trying something else new in the coming weeks. Research what else is available locally or online – try one new form of exercise in the next month and see how it makes you feel. Is it something that you could add to your list of enjoyable ways to move your body?

Food Shopping Trip

Make food shopping joyful by seeking out a local food market and visiting somewhere new for fresh produce, making an outing of it. Suggest a meet-up with friends at a farmer's market or similar and help a small local business while buying fresh produce and food items. You could make it a once-a-month activity with friends.

Find your Sanctuary

Create a space in your home where you can rest and not be disturbed when you need to take some time for yourself. It could be just a corner of your bedroom, or a space in your garden – you want it to feel relaxing, indulgent and positive.

Also look at your sleeping space and declutter it so that the room feels airy, in order and restful. You don't want work items or "to-do" piles in there getting in the way of you being able to switch off and relax.

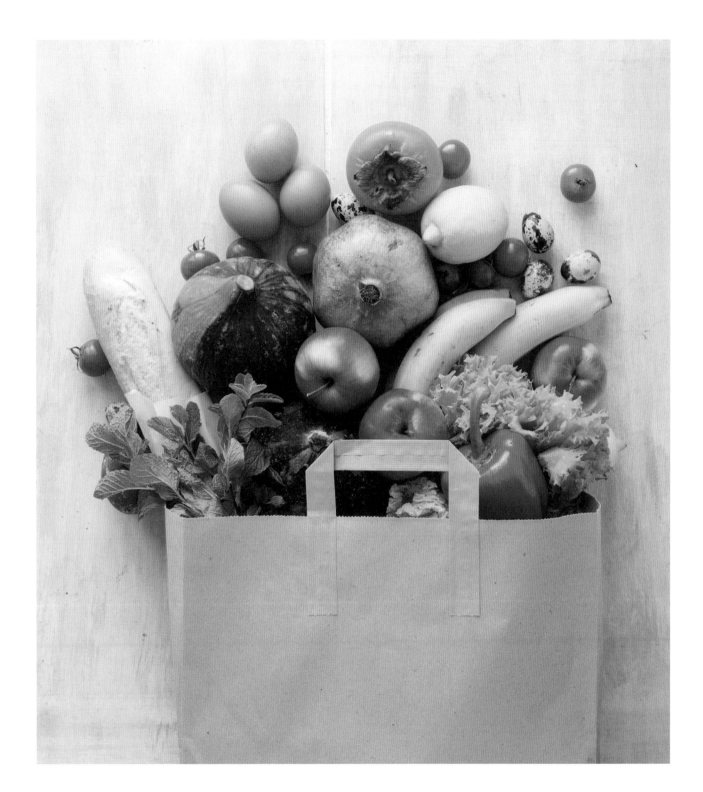

DAY 19

Salsa

This dance is all about rhythm and hips. I always think of salsa as a little bit cheeky and I find it helps when I'm doing a salsa routine to put on a skirt so I feel something moving around as I dance. It's amazing what a little change of costume can do for your fun levels. With this one, try to get in as much hip action as possible. It doesn't matter if your hips are going the wrong way, just enjoy moving your body in that figure 8 motion. Put the music on and get stuck in.

Warm-up: Curtsy Squats x 10 on each side

- Basic Step x 16
- Basic Side-step x 16
- Zulu x 8
- Spot Turn x 1
- Repeat 2–4 times

Cool down: Plié Squat with arms overhead and hold for 20 seconds, or however long feels good

Exercise Challenge

I want you to look forward and set yourself a fun exercise challenge for the month ahead. I'm not talking about a marathon or climbing a mountain – but look at what's resonated with you and worked for you these past weeks, and what you've enjoyed. Maybe you could aim to master three new salsa or tap steps. Perhaps you should research local park runs if you think that you'd like to dust off your running shoes. What about a skipping challenge for the month?

Also, why not set yourself a challenge to try a form of exercise that you've never tried before – Ju Jitsu, open swimming or ballroom dancing are all ways to combine a hobby with movement, socialize and have fun.

Dinner Date

Invite some people over for breakfast, lunch or dinner to trial a new dish or ingredient, and to share a new taste. Enjoying the food you're making is so important and doing so with loved ones is even better. Use the meal as an inspiration to try something new or share a dish you've found and loved.

A Self-Care Day

There is nothing better than taking a self-care day for yourself, it feels totally amazing! Rather than a random half hour here or there, aim for a full day – put it in your diary now and start planning for it. If taking a full day off is difficult, take 30 minutes today to do something entirely for yourself. Can you put this in your diary as a twice-weekly event? Remember that when you put self-care first, you encourage those around you to do the same – spreading that good feeling and setting expectations that you are making yourself a priority. Putting an effort into healthy self-care habits repeatedly really pays off.

"Enjoying the food you're making is so important and doing so with loved ones is even better."

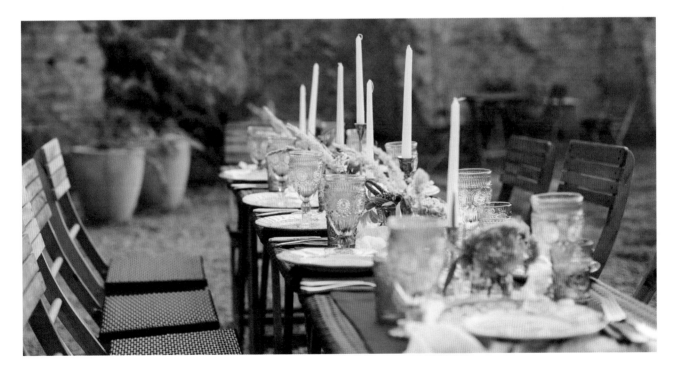

DAY 20

Yoga for Balance

Obviously in dancing, I need good balance and the core is crucial for this. But balance work is also good for the mind as it takes a lot of focus, so it's exercising your mind as well as using your core and legs. Learning how to focus to engage your balance is the key learning here.

Warm-up: standing Knee to Chest on both sides for 3–5 breaths

- Tree Pose on right leg for 3–5 breaths
- High Lunge with Twist Variation, right leg forward for 3–5 breaths
- Side Plank with left hand on floor for 3–5 breaths. Bonus: try the Lifting Leg Variation for an additional 3–5 breaths
- High Lunge, right leg forward for 3–5 breaths
- Warrior 3, right leg forward for 3–5 breaths
- Right Knee to Chest in standing position for 3–5 breaths
- Repeat the routine on the left side

Cool down: Knee to Chest on both sides for 30–60 seconds, or however long feels good

Favourite Routines

We're not finished yet, but today is a good time to consider what you would pick for your top three desert island exercise routines. Ask yourself why they make you happy. What is it about the routine that works for you – how does it make you feel? Is it quick and easy? Is it good for stretching your body? Does it make time pass quickly?

Look for answers to guide you for your exercise going forward.

Back to School

Why not sign up for a cookery course to try something new or learn a new skill? It's a great way to gain hands-on tips and extra confidence. There are courses available in everything from cooking authentic curries to foraging and cheese-making to cooking for special diets. It's also another really social way to learn more about food.

Visualization Board

Now that you've had nearly three weeks to examine and think about how to build time for your personal priorities, I want you to look ahead at your short-term and long-term goals. How do you want to feel more of the time? What does the new you look like? What do you wear? How do you feel? Use your answers to create a visualization board for the year ahead (see page 45–6). What are your joyful goals? Focus on specific aims and the small steps to get you to where you want to be.

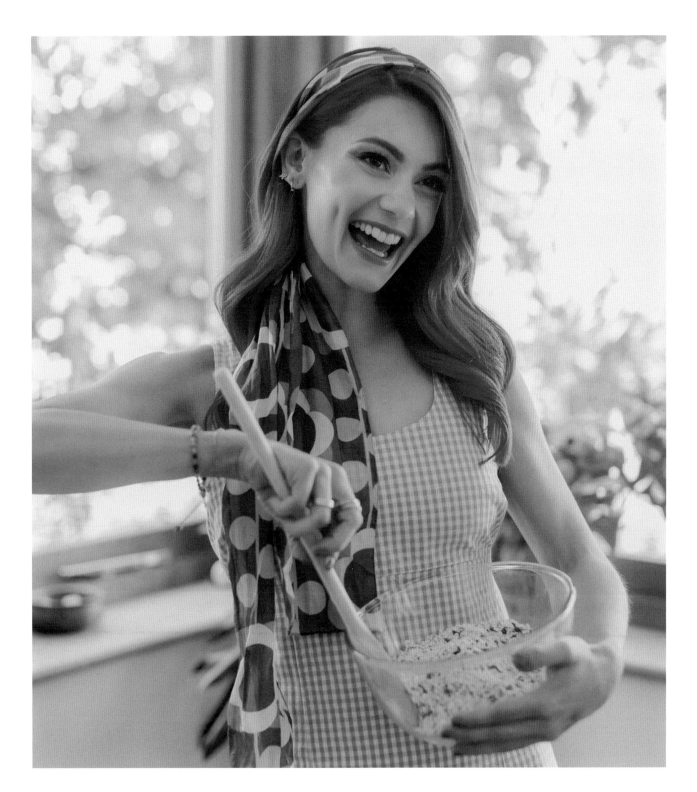

DAY 21

Short Sun Salutation

For me, this routine is something I do before I'm about to dance or do a show as it's a lovely warm-up for the body for any form of exercise. It gives you some fire in the belly – I call it my little "fire belly warm-up."

You've probably come across a Sun Salutation if you've done any yoga as it often starts a class. It's a short series of stretches (originally for a ceremonial role) that calms and focuses the mind. What's not to love?

Remember that the flowing movement from one pose to the next should be done in conjunction with the breath – either on an inhale or an exhale. Try to hold each pose for 3–5 breaths.

- Mountain Pose into
- Forward Fold into
- Halfway Lift into
- Straight Arm Plank into
- Upward Dog into
- Downward Dog into
- Low Lunge into
- Halfway Lift into
- Mountain Pose
- Repeat the routine on both sides 3–4 times

What are your Exercise Goals?

Twenty-one days down and it's both time to congratulate yourself for all you've achieved these past three weeks and to think about what comes next. This is a fantastic start, and now you get to decide what to do with this new knowledge, skill and determination. Where is your joyful exercise going to take you next? I'm excited for you.

What are your Nutrition Goals?

Take some time to have a look back at what's changed with your eating habits over the past three weeks. Do you feel different in your body for trying different foods and increasing healthy wholefoods? Certain foods don't work for everyone – our bodies are all different and learning what suits your body is key to finding healthy ways to enjoy food. What is great though is variety and maxing out the healthy options that help make our body stronger and more energized.

Gold Medal Winner

Consider today your winner's ceremony for everything you've achieved these past weeks. Reflect on the successes you've had in the 21 days. What are the best things you've got out of the plan? What wins the award for best new habit, new favourite app or best new food discovery? Be proud of your achievements.

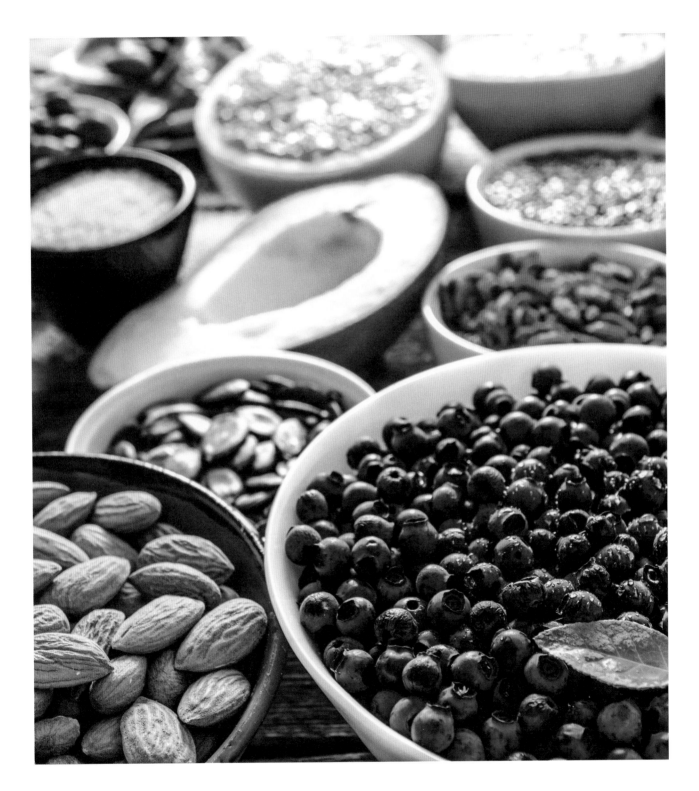

WHAT NEXT?

Now you're at the end of your 21-day adventure and I hope you are excited about the changes you're seeing in body and mind. I'm sure there have been good days and bad, easy days and hard. I'd love to hear from you about the most significant differences you've noticed – perhaps you feel in a much better mood, you have more energy, your clothes are looser, you are more focused, have a more flexible body or maybe you're feeling a lot more confident about yourself. Whatever your age or level of fitness, and whatever your reasons for doing this plan, you'll feel the effects of the endorphins as your movement increases. Moving your body more makes you feel at your best.

If you've enjoyed these past three weeks, it's time to make the effort to keep the habit going. Why not look into other forms of exercise? Did you enjoy netball at school? Do you yearn to strap on roller boots again? Paddleboarding doesn't feel the same as going to the gym, but it's actually a really brilliant way to move your body and get out in nature, and if you enjoy it then you're motivated to do it regularly (rather than the five times a year many gym goers manage). Hiking up a mountain or walking in a forest is the same – immersing yourself in beautiful nature while you move your body gives you the double whammy of a mental and physical health boost. If you loved some of the routines these past weeks, then find a local group or sign up for some online classes and try that style of exercise again. Or commit to a fitness challenge with a friend. And don't forget to grab five minutes at the start or end of every day for a quick stretch routine, or to put on some music and jive or tap until your heart is pumping hard.

The important thing is to enjoy yourself and make the most of your time. Get moving and get happy!

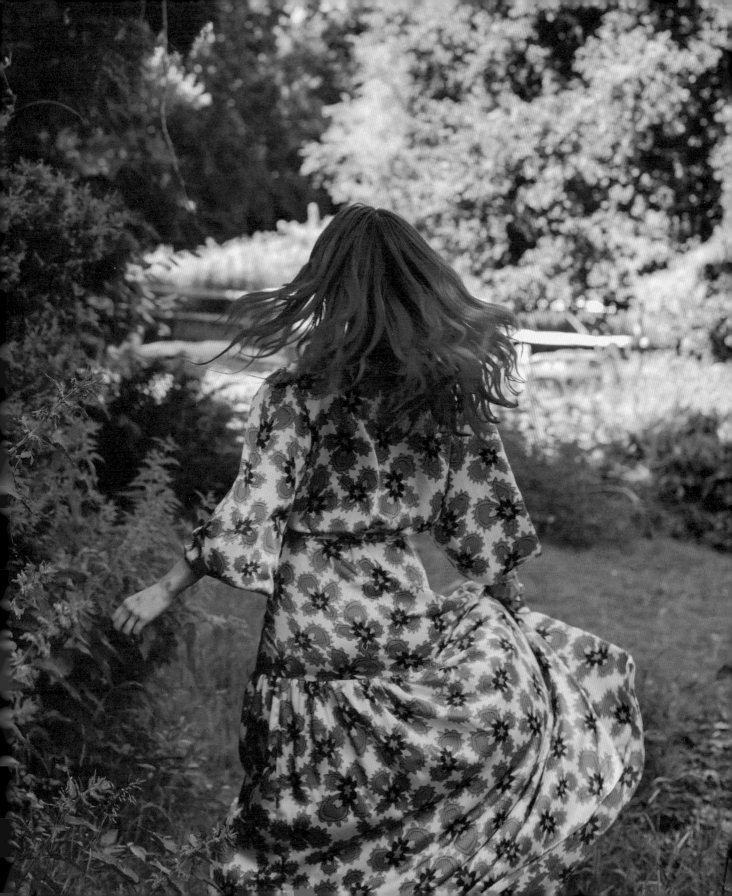

ACKNOWLEDGEMENTS

Thank you to Joe Sugg for being my biggest supporter and believing in everything I do. Thanks also to Liv Russo at Margravine, who has been there every step of the way through this journey. Thank you to Kate Latham, who helped me to bring my thoughts and ideas to life, and to Katrina Lipska from Kat's Films for taking such wonderful photos. Finally, thank you to the entire team at Watkins Publishing for believing in me and this book.

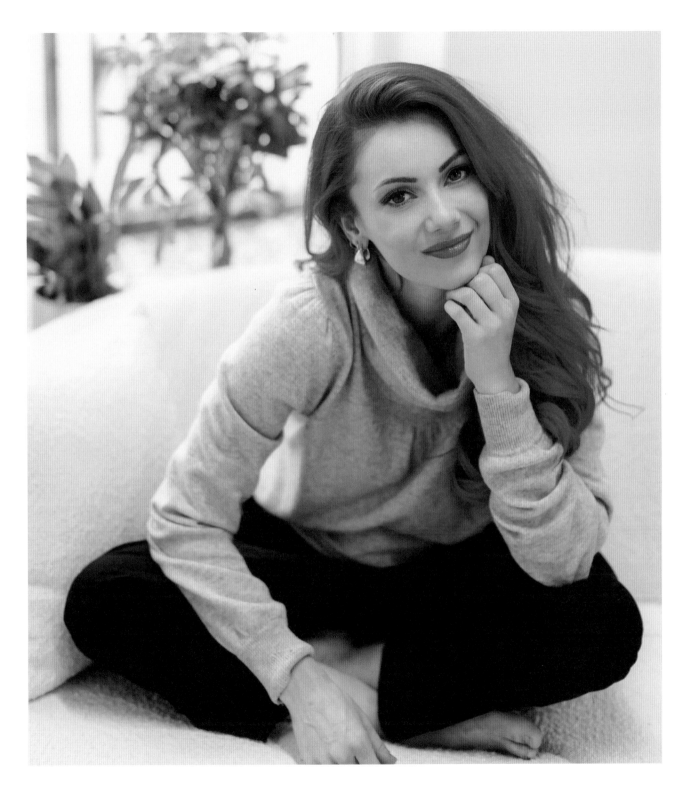

ACKNOWLEDGEMENTS
205

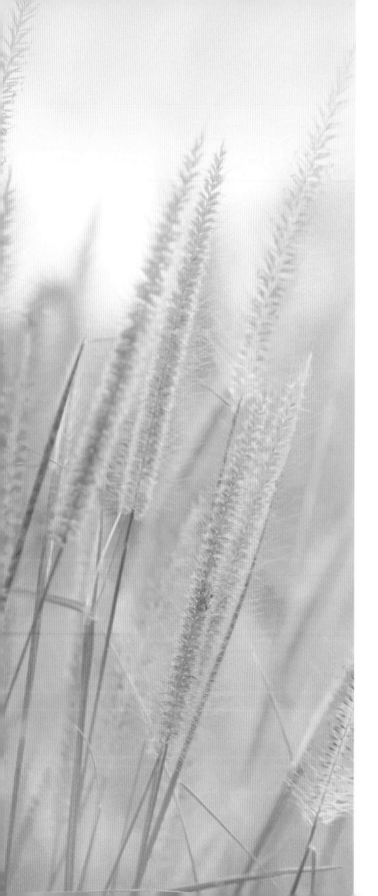

INDEX

WATKINS
Sharing Wisdom
Since 1893

The story of Watkins began in 1893, when scholar of esotericism John Watkins founded our bookshop, inspired by the lament of his friend and teacher Madame Blavatsky that there was nowhere in London to buy books on mysticism, occultism or metaphysics. That moment marked the birth of Watkins, soon to become the publisher of many of the leading lights of spiritual literature, including Carl Jung, Rudolf Steiner, Alice Bailey and Chögyam Trungpa.

Today, the passion at Watkins Publishing for vigorous questioning is still resolute. Our stimulating and groundbreaking list ranges from ancient traditions and complementary medicine to the latest ideas about personal development, holistic wellbeing and consciousness exploration. We remain at the cutting edge, committed to publishing books that change lives.

DISCOVER MORE AT:
www.watkinspublishing.com

Read our blog

Watch and listen to our authors in action

Sign up to our mailing list

We celebrate conscious, passionate, wise and happy living.
Be part of that community by visiting

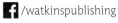 /watkinspublishing   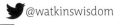 @watkinswisdom

/watkinsbooks   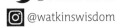 @watkinswisdom